INTENSIVE CARE

GAVIN FRANCIS has worked across four continents as a surgeon, emergency physician, medical officer with the British Antarctic Survey and latterly as a GP; he has described the pandemic response of 2020–21 as the most intense period of his twenty-year career in medicine. He's the author of the *Sunday Times* bestseller *Adventures in Human Being*, which was a BMA Book of the Year, and *Shapeshifters*. His books have won the SMIT Scottish Book of the Year Award and the Saltire Award for Non-Fiction, and have been shortlisted for the Ondaatje and Costa Prizes. He also writes for the *Guardian*, *The Times*, the ~~London Review~~ of *Books* and *Granta*. He lives in Edinb~~urgh~~

D1390961

wellcome
collection

WELLCOME COLLECTION publishes thought-provoking books exploring health and human experience, in partnership with leading independent publisher Profile Books.

WELLCOME COLLECTION is a free museum and library that aims to challenge how we think and feel about health by connecting science, medicine, life and art, through exhibitions, collections, live programming, and more. It is part of Wellcome, a global charitable foundation that supports science to solve urgent health challenges, with a focus on mental health, infectious diseases and climate.

wellcomecollection.org

INTENSIVE CARE

A GP, A COMMUNITY & A PANDEMIC

GAVIN FRANCIS

This paperback edition first published in 2021

First published in Great Britain in 2021 by
Profile Books Ltd
29 Cloth Fair
London
EC1A 7JQ
www.profilebooks.com

Published in association with Wellcome Collection

**wellcome
collection**

183 Euston Road
London NW1 2BE
www.wellcomecollection.org

Printed and bound in Great Britain by
CPI Group (UK) Ltd, Croydon, CR0 4YY

A CIP catalogue record for this book is available from the British Library.

ISBN 978 1 78816 733 8
eISBN 978 1 78283 816 6

For carers of all kinds
(for the kindness of carers)

A NOTE ON CONFIDENTIALITY

This book takes the reader into the coronavirus pandemic as seen beyond the walls of the hospital, out in the communities that I work with, and for, urban and rural.

Just as physicians must honour the privileged access they have to our bodies, they must honour the trust with which we share our stories. As a doctor who is also a writer, I've spent a great deal of time deliberating over what can and cannot be said without betraying the confidence of my patients.

The reflections that follow are all grounded in events within my clinical experience, but the patients in them have been so disguised as to be unrecognisable – any similarities that remain are coincidental. Protecting confidences is an essential part of what I do: 'confidence' means 'with faith' – we are all patients sooner or later; we all want faith that we'll be heard, and that our privacy will be respected.

Contents

INTRODUCTION

*'[I]t is my opinion, and I must leave it as a prescription, viz.,
that the best physic against the plague is to run away from it.'*
Daniel Defoe
A Journal of the Plague Year

At the Covid clinic car park the barrier points skywards: the
requirement to pay is suspended, along with so many other
rules in this strange, in-between world of coronavirus. The
clinic doctors had told you to come alone. You walk to the
door, breathless even at that brief exertion, then push a
buzzer that will shortly be wiped with alcohol to decontami-
nate it from your touch. You wait, with your cough and your
fever. The door opens; inside, a nurse in blue scrubs, face
mask and visor helps you put on a face mask, then leads you
down the red or 'dirty' corridor (though it is decorated in
pastel shades and looks freshly mopped) into a small clinic
room with too-bright lights and wipe-down furniture. You're
gasping now for breath, have some pains in your chest, you're
flushed and sweating, frightened by all you've heard and read
of this virus, this pandemic. The millions downed by it, the
lack of ventilators, the military drafted in to help, the global
economic ruin.

A doctor comes in; she too is dressed in impersonal blue
scrubs, a mask with a spray visor, a flimsy plastic apron and
bare forearms ending in blue-gloved hands. She asks you a
few questions – how breathless you feel, how high your fever
has been, when did your symptoms start, where you have
been travelling. She puts a sensor on your finger to gauge the

1

oxygen content of your blood, then slots a thermometer into your ear. You feel hungry for air, and notice her gaze on you, as she counts your breaths.

Your oxygen is too low, your breathing too fast; a wheelchair is brought, a porter takes you to a lift. You still have your mask on and when, inside the lift, you ask the porter where you're going, his own mask makes it difficult to understand the response. The lift door opens, behind it more blue-suited figures dressed in masks, aprons and gloves. One approaches with a swab on a stick, but you can't make out clearly what is said. You feel swallowed by the hospital, by the virus, by this pandemic that has broken over the world.

This story begins on 31 December 2019 when the Chinese authorities alerted the World Health Organization (WHO) to a new and dangerous strain of viral pneumonia that had arisen in Wuhan, central China. That virus didn't yet have a name, though it had already been circulating for some months. As the world turned into a new year, midnight fireworks igniting in a band across the globe, the virus began its worldwide spread. The story of 2020 is the story of this virus, its transmission, its ramifications for global and local economies, for how we travel, how we deliver healthcare, and how we plan for the even more damaging epidemics that will come.

My ambition has been to chart the evolution of this modern epidemic as I saw it, as a GP and as a member of the communities I work with, and for, in Scotland. In fact, the story that I am telling has proven more complex, and its ramifications more extended, than I anticipated in the early weeks of the crisis. Back then my fear was of a deluge of infections and deaths caused by the virus. I didn't see that this would become not just an account of a pandemic infection, but of the sudden warping of an entire way of life, of all those lives which have been thrown out of kilter and whose trajectories were now so uncertain, and the care those people would need as a result. I didn't foresee how much the profession that I love would be bruised, transformed and reshaped to cope with the impact of the virus. This book is a contemporary history, an eyewitness account of the most intense months I have known in my twenty-year career, a hot take on the pandemic that speaks of the tragic consequences of measures taken against the virus as much as it tells stories of the virus itself.

'Crisis' is a Greek word which originally described the moment in the evolution of an illness on which everything hinges, when death and recovery are held, for a moment, in the balance. The slightest nudge towards one or the other may determine the outcome. In a hospital, the intensive care unit or intensive therapy unit (ICU or ITU) is where the sickest patients, those whose organs are failing and who will die without drastic and intense interventions, are looked after. Those units do extraordinary work, but over the months of this pandemic it has often seemed to me as if many other clinicians, scientists, carers and charity workers outside the ITU have been engaged in something comparably intense. It has frequently seemed as if society itself is on life support, and intensive measures, including huge efforts of selflessness, vision and compassion, have been required to sustain it. 'Care' is something we do for others, but it's also an emotional attitude of attentive compassion, of kindness, and delivering it can be a privilege as much as it can also be a burden and a responsibility. I'd like to cast a modest spotlight on the care I've seen delivered in the communities I work with – a care that has often been delivered quietly, without headline news, in rural village streets, community clinics and communal city stairs. It's my hope that sharing some of those stories will help readers see more clearly what has been gained and lost so far through Covid-19, and what we're still in danger of losing. It's only by learning from this pandemic that we can better protect ourselves for the next one.

PART I

ESCALATION

INCUBATION

'[T]he infection was propagated insensibly, and by such persons as were not visibly infected, who neither knew whom they infected or who they were infected by.'
Daniel Defoe
A Journal of the Plague Year

On 13 January 2020 a bulletin from Health Protection Scotland was sent to all GP practices in the country describing a 'novel Wuhan coronavirus'. I work in a small clinic in central Edinburgh with four doctors, two nurses and six admin staff, responsible for almost 4,000 patients. It was the first time I'd heard of the virus. 'Current reports describe no evidence of significant human to human transmission, including no infections of healthcare workers,' the note said, reassuringly.

I cast my mind back to the SARS coronavirus of almost two decades ago, now referred to as SARS-CoV-1, and briefly wondered how quickly the spread of this coronavirus would be stopped, as that one was. A seafood market had been closed and sanitised. The bulletin said that although Wuhan was a city of 19 million people, there were only three flights per week from there to the UK, and the likely impact was 'Very Low'. I gave it a moment's thought, then carried on with my work.

Scientists had already discovered that the new virus was

different from SARS-CoV-1, though still within the family of coronaviruses. These were first seen under the electron microscope in 1964 by a Scottish virologist, June Almeida, in a sample swabbed from a boy with symptoms of the common cold. 'Corona' refers to the spiky little packets of sugared protein stuck all over the surface of the spherical virus, like fleurs-de-lys sprouting from the band of a crown, or the flared corona of the sun. Under an electron microscope they look like tiny planets, each one buzzing with angry satellites. It's been estimated that between 5 per cent and 10 per cent of common colds are caused by coronaviruses of one kind or another – they're a perennial nuisance to human populations, and usually cause mild illness. SARS-CoV-1, though, was more severe in its effects (hence the name 'Severe Acute Respiratory Syndrome'): between 2002 and 2003 it infected about 8,000 people across 29 countries, causing almost 800 deaths.

Coronaviruses are a similar size to flu viruses – 0.1 microns in diameter – and are widespread among many different mammals. SARS-CoV-1 came to humans from the Asian civet; Middle East Respiratory Syndrome (MERS), which emerged in 2012 and caused the deaths of around 2,500 people (mostly in Saudi Arabia), came via dromedary camels. The new virus had its origin in bats, but whether there was another mammalian intermediary between bats and humans was, at the time I was reading the bulletin, uncertain.

I spent the afternoon of 13 January in the library of the Royal College of Physicians on Edinburgh's Queen Street – it is Scotland's oldest medical library, containing some 60,000 volumes, some going back to the 1400s. It's a calm place to study and write, with windows that face north over the trees and gardens of the city's New Town and the Firth of Forth. Later that evening I met up with a friend, a consultant physician who'd recently come back to clinical work after a period of time doing research. She was stationed at a general hospital thirty miles or so from Edinburgh, and was enjoying being back in the thick of it, though startled at how stretched her medical colleagues were. The annual winter flu season was on us, and beds in hospital were tight. 'It's the same every year,' she said. 'I wonder when health boards will realise how many winter beds we actually need.'

A week later, Chinese infections stood at 550, and the death toll: 17. A new bulletin arrived reassuring me that the risk of infection was still low, but attaching a form to be completed should I suspect someone of having the virus – specifically anyone flying in from Wuhan. My practice looks after hundreds of students; I was disgruntled but not alarmed when one of the Edinburgh universities asked worried Chinese students to seek their GP's attention. 'By phone!' I wanted them to add. 'Tell them to seek attention by phone!'

Meanwhile Zhong Nanshan, head of the Chinese National Health Commission's team investigating the virus, confirmed that it was not constrained to spreading through infected animals, but could spread between infected humans. There were two people ill with the virus who had caught it from family members and fourteen healthcare workers were confirmed as having fallen ill through caring for infected patients. China was in the thick of the Lunar Holiday season – the time of year in which the greatest number of journeys within China are made – 2 billion trips. Millions of journeys are also made between China and the rest of the world for the same holiday. Countries in east Asia, nervous about the virus and primed by memories of SARS-CoV-1, began to screen arrivals from China for fever, asking them about cough symptoms.

By 24 January train and plane journeys from Wuhan and nearby Xiantao and Chibi were all cancelled. The WHO said they had, at that time, no evidence of human to human spread outside of China. More cities around Wuhan in Hubei province closed down, putting the number of people under quarantine at around 40 million.

In Scotland, 25 January is celebrated as the birthday of the poet Robert Burns: I had invitations to Burns suppers that weekend in Edinburgh, and with friends I joined crowds walking between film installations projected on to some of the city's most famous public buildings, visuals accompanied by poetry and music. Close to the city centre, Robin Robertson's poem 'Ten Thousand Miles Of Edge' illuminated a monument on Calton Hill. We stood high on the hill, the lights of the city beneath us like raked embers, the darkness of the river Forth to the north and, beyond it, the coastline of Fife diminishing as it merged with the North Sea, listening to Robertson's voice: low, wry, grave and severe, reading 'the sea protects us, the sea links us'.

That weekend celebratory events for Chinese New Year were cancelled in Beijing and the first death outside Hubei province was reported. Five more cities locked down, a hard-to-imagine 56 million people affected. Dinner in Edinburgh that night at a friend's house was haggis, neeps and tatties washed down with a half bottle of whisky. We discussed the virus, but briefly: there was still the sense that this problem was a distant one, something for east Asia to deal with; perhaps a few flailing sparks of infection might need to be extinguished elsewhere. But it was all in hand, it would be fixed, and the planet would go on twisting into the sun each morning and we'd keep our usual concerns: Brexit, politics, ageing, the changing climate.

The word 'epidemic' is Greek and means 'upon the people'; it carries the sense of a burden endured – a concise way of describing the oppressive fear of infectious outbreaks in the centuries before anyone had any idea of the bacteria and viruses that cause them. There was no distinction, then, between such disparate areas of knowledge as medicine, meteorology, natural science and nutrition. The first writings on the subject have a startling breadth as to what might have a bearing on the rampant spread of disease. 'There was much rain in Thasos about the time of the autumnal equinox' begins the *Epidemics* of Hippocrates. 'It fell gently and continuously and the wind was from the south ... but the spring was cold with southerly winds and there was little rain.'

Reading between the lines, you can feel the frustration of these early physicians, oblivious of the rudiments of infection control, casting around for some way of understanding the devastation inflicted on their patients. Respiratory infections like coronavirus and influenza were undoubtedly known to the physicians collectively known as 'Hippocrates', one of whom wrote of a plague in Greece in Book 1 of the *Epidemics*, around 400 BCE. 'Many patients had dry, unproductive coughs and hoarse voices ... Some had fever, but not all.' Later in the same book another plague is described: 'of those who contracted it death was most common among youths, young men, men in the prime of life ... those with thin voices, those with rough voices.' Perhaps those Greek physicians were on to something – it's since been found there *is* an association between the severity of a respiratory illness and alterations to the voice. In later months, I would read in a daily news bulletin of artificial intelligence research seeking a vocal signature of coronavirus, using voice sampling from smartphones.

In some ways epidemics remain as bewildering and burdensome to us now as they have been at any time in the history of humanity. But in truth we understand immeasurably more about them, and have, in theory, the knowledge to limit their spread (though with Covid-19, it's conspicuous how much we failed to put this knowledge into action).

The book of Genesis speaks of waves of plague breaking over Egypt; in 430 BCE there was an epidemic in Athens that killed a quarter of the population (like Covid-19, its symptoms included 'headache, coughing, chest pains'). About 5 million people are thought to have died in the Antonine Plague (probably smallpox) of the Roman Empire, and in the mid-200s CE a plague in Rome was killing 5,000 citizens a day.

Looking back through history, it's easy – or it was, at least, in January – to pity our ancestors, at the mercy of forces they barely understood, and awash in misinformation. Epidemics were once thought to wax and wane at the whim of the gods or the heavens, and the word 'influenza' derives from the perceived 'influence' of the stars. But they've also long been associated with a more familiar series of changes: the flux of the seasons. 'In all cases so far described,' wrote Hippocrates, 'the spring was the worst time and most of the deaths occurred then; the summer was the easiest time and few died then ... For the coming of winter terminates summer diseases, and the coming of summer shifts winter diseases.'

Compare this with a World Health Organization statement on the novel Wuhan coronavirus: 'Currently the northern hemisphere (and China) is in the midst of the winter season when Influenza and other respiratory infections are prevalent ... countries need to take into consideration that travellers with signs and symptoms suggestive of respiratory infection may result from respiratory diseases other than Covid-19.' In other words, when it comes to epidemics, seasons matter as much now as they ever did.

*

On 29 January the first cases of the new coronavirus were confirmed in the UK: a Chinese couple staying in a hotel in York. The following day, 30 January, the WHO announced a global health emergency as the death toll reached 170 in China, and the cases in that country alone reached almost 8,000. Cases were also confirmed in India and the Philippines.

I also received my first instruction to tell patients to 'self-isolate' even if they had no symptoms. It was from Lothian NHS Board, and asked that anyone coming from Wuhan city lock themselves away for fourteen days, even if they had no symptoms. They were to

> inform NHS 24 of their travel history and symptoms when they call. If they become symptomatic they should not leave their home until they have been given advice by a clinician. That coronaviruses do not usually spread if people don't have symptoms, but we cannot be 100% sure – so this is a precautionary measure.

This would later be shown to be wrong – one of the reasons SARS-CoV-2 is so devastatingly effective as a virus is its ability to spread without triggering symptoms of illness. The instructions also informed us that masks 'and other personal protective equipment' would be sent to us shortly. We didn't have a great deal of faith in NHS procurement, particularly for workers in general practice, and the instruction prompted jokes among my colleagues that we'd be sent a paper bag and some of those cling film gloves you get at petrol stations. But we were wrong: some surgical masks did arrive later that week, and tear-off plastic aprons.

During the week I work at my small Edinburgh practice, but at the weekend I work evening shifts at an 'out of hours'

(OOH) centre in the city covering a much larger population, with a different team of doctors and nurses. I had an email from the clinical director of the centre, Sian Tucker, advising me to tell any patients from mainland China outside Wuhan that they would only need to self-isolate if they had symptoms, adding that those symptoms did *not* include a sore throat. Until then I'd been assuming that a dripping nose and a sore throat would be the herald of coronavirus infection, the way those symptoms are the manifestation of most respiratory viruses. My practice started a WhatsApp group to keep one another updated. It proved as helpful for sharing joke videos as for divesting the latest governmental advice.

In my routine clinic in Edinburgh's city centre, Monday to Friday, my three colleagues and I began slowly to orientate ourselves towards the changes this virus might make necessary. I had worked as a GP for fifteen years, having moved to that role after six years in hospital medicine focussing on surgery and on emergency medicine. I was drawn to general practice for the way its work is balanced between clinic and home visits, young and old, the mundane and the life-threatening. There are many things to love about the work: the variety of different encounters with people who flow through the clinic doors each day, the breadth of their concerns, the intimacy of the private consulting space with its ethical codes of confidentiality and candour, the strange mingling of science and kindness, the intuitive leaps made necessary by the constraints of time and resources. The work is satisfying because it is, at its heart, about listening to people's stories and offering modest, practical advice.

Strictly speaking, UK general practice clinics are not part of the NHS; they're small businesses run by the doctors who are for the most part 'partners' rather than employees. But they're odd businesses, in that they have essentially only one customer: the National Health Service, which 'buys' healthcare for a defined population, paying each practice through a complex and historically convoluted set of mechanisms that have somehow stood through seven decades with only minor adjustments. The distinction of being theoretically independent brings freedom, autonomy and agility, but it also brings administrative hassles and money concerns that pass hospital specialists by: surgeons aren't obliged to own and maintain their operating theatres the way many GPs have to own and maintain their surgery premises, for example.

Just as the funding mechanisms of general practice hadn't changed much in seventy years, so too the model to which many of us worked: a reception, a waiting room, a series of clinical offices in which each doctor spent two or three hours in the morning, and again in the afternoon, seeing between twelve and sixteen people and talking to them about their problems, one after the other, in short, often pre-arranged appointments. At busy times the waiting room would be full, and for flu jab clinics in the autumn the corridors would be crammed as, between us, the doctors and nurses of the practice would vaccinate about a quarter of the practice population in the space of a few weeks – those whose age or infirmity meant they were more susceptible than the wider population.

Lunch was often skipped or hurried, the time between morning and afternoon clinics filled with home visits, and with reading volumes of correspondence from hospital colleagues: advice; letters on anyone who'd been recently discharged from hospital; reports on X-rays and ultrasound scans; results of blood tests we'd taken ourselves; summaries of specialist reviews on everything from audiology to urology. Some doctors find reading through correspondence a chore, but it has never felt like that to me: diagnosing illness can feel like being set a series of intricate and cryptic puzzles, and reading correspondence from specialists can be like turning to the back page solutions. There's satisfaction in having my questions answered and, when no answers are forthcoming, there's a comfort in knowing that sometimes even an expert trained for thirty years in their chosen organ or disease can be as baffled by a patient's symptoms as I am. Doctors are far more fallible in their judgements and their diagnostic abilities than they are usually prepared to admit.

After reading the correspondence I'd make a few telephone calls to people who simply wanted my advice, or whose correspondence had thrown up anomalies and questions that needed resolution or a change in treatment: an alteration in antibiotic for one; a reduction in the dose of water pills or blood pressure meds for another. Then, after that, it was out on my bike, not in Lycra but in smart trousers tucked into my socks and often, given the Edinburgh weather, waterproofs, visiting people too frail or fearful to be able to manage to visit the GP practice itself. In slums and in mansions, in high-rise apartments and disability-adapted bungalows, GP work offers insights into how people really live in ways that many hospital colleagues envy. On a home visit I'm acutely aware that I'm not on my home turf, but invited into someone else's space – that invitation shifts the dynamic of the medical encounter in subtle but powerful ways, towards the patient's agenda and away from the doctor's.

31 January, a typical Friday. The first patient is a 4-week-old baby, a third child, who's apparently been screaming the house down but is tranquil now. Screaming for babies of course isn't unusual, but there's a harshness to the cry, and the mother, being experienced, has been alarmed by it. There

must be something wrong, she says. The baby vomits, too, that's new, and every time she starts screaming a bulge appears in her side. Where? I ask. There, I can show you. She takes out her phone and plays me a video, and there on the crystal screen I can see the bulge appear with each scream. As I watch I place my hand on the infant's belly, pushing gently, trying to feel through the skin with my fingertips towards the baby's tiny pebble kidneys, the convex spleen, intestines as thin as bullrushes. But I can't feel anything untoward. The baby is tranquil, feeding from her mother – such peace some spend their whole lives trying to rediscover – and I know that in seconds she will be screaming as if disembowelled again, and that mysterious swelling will rise again from her side. She needs an ultrasound scan of the belly, and I speak to the paediatricians to arrange it.

Next a man in his eighties, a retired schoolteacher who always wears a tie to our visits. He'd fallen and cracked a bone in his back. He's sorry to trouble me, but could I just help him with his pain, with the side-effects of the painkillers, with advice on how long the healing will take? In a conversation of courtly politeness we circle the plastic skeleton that hangs in my consulting room, discussing the anatomy of the spine. Then a woman of late middle age who couldn't hold on to her urine; the exercises I'd suggested were 'useless' and a brief trial of drugs had desiccated her mouth. An ultrasound scan of her bladder, when full and when empty, had added nothing, and I referred her for consideration of surgery to her pelvic muscles. A woman of twenty scratching at her skin – she had picked up scabies from a flatmate. A girl whose mother said she had food intolerances; from her bag she pulled a colour-coded list three pages in length, grouped together by symptoms and food groups, and asked me to go through it with her. A man whose birthday it was that day: ninety years! A tiny avatar of a cake with candles had appeared in the bottom left corner of my screen. At my congratulations he beamed, told me he'd meet his grandchildren for lunch, and I went back to explaining the purpose of all the new medications he'd been given since his stroke. A 50-year-old archaeologist, a badminton enthusiast who wore a beard like Trotsky and whose shoulder injury hadn't settled despite three months of physiotherapy. With a long, sterile needle I breached the hidden space between his shoulderblade and humerus, and injected a vial-full of steroids. A 6-year-old with tonsillitis, who opened her mouth for my inspection with the enthusiasm of a hippo having its teeth cleaned. A 92-year-old retired postmistress with memory loss, together with her son; every example of forgetfulness the son offered was forcefully denied by the mother, with a pout of indignation; together the son and I coaxed her towards accepting a formal assessment at a memory clinic, and a CT scan of her brain. A 74-year-old widow, a retired lollipop lady, unsteady on her feet. A fifty-something nurse with a chest infection. A feverish toddler who lay in her mother's arms, blotchy and panting, having vomited up her breakfast. She watched me with malevolent distrust as I pushed on her belly, testing for pain. A man in his sixties with chronic depression, his face demolished by age and sadness. That was the morning clinic over with.

There were three phone calls: to check in on a marketing executive who'd been measuring his own blood pressure at home; to a woman whom I'd been treating for joint pains, to see if her tablets were working; and to a young man who'd been cutting himself – the psychiatrists had recommended mood stabilisers, and I was relieved to hear that they'd been helping.

Then three home visits: to a woman recovering from breast cancer surgery, who lived alone and isolated in a high-rise apartment, and who before her surgery rarely left the home. From her window we looked out over the city, its industry and traffic, the windows catching brief shafts of sunlight, each building shining like a cage of light. The second was to a care home which was once a baronial mansion. I locked my bike to a tree trunk in the garden and rang its bell, then was led by a Filipina nurse to see my patient, Miss Nicol. She'd been refusing food and lashing out at the care staff. I watched as the nurse, Nenita, succeeded with great skill in calming her, then coaxed her to accept sips of water and her medications. Miss Nicol was aged 94 and the survivor of many years of dementia; her closest relative, a nephew, lived in Australia. As I examined her with care, trying not to provoke her, I remembered an afternoon the previous summer when the nephew, in Scotland for a holiday, came to my clinic to talk about his aunt. 'No heroics,' he'd told me, 'she always said she couldn't bear to depend on anyone, and now look at her.' I told Nenita I had little to add, and that if Miss Nicol wouldn't eat, I didn't think we should oblige her to, and we certainly shouldn't admit her to hospital. Many conscientious and caring nursing home staff have a fear of being accused of neglect, so being able to document 'no action' after medical review meant that Nenita and her colleagues could get on with doing what they were so good at: caring for this old lady with dignity, in a place she knew well.

The third visit of the day was to a woman dying of a brain tumour who couldn't walk, whose forefeet had swollen up like toadstools, and whose stomach had been bleeding from the inside. There's a mysterious connection between the brain and the stomach as if the belly reacts in sympathy to any trauma endured by the head (it's not unusual for the victims of severe head injury to develop stomach ulcers). Now the swelling in the woman's head that threatened to blind her, that was slowly paralysing her limbs, had released some haemorrhage of the gut. I began to think that perhaps she wouldn't die of the tumour after all, but of bleeding. I started speaking to her gently, watching her expression, talking of patients I'd known in the past who'd reached this advanced stage of cancer, who'd tired of hospitals and who couldn't bear the thought of being processed through their bureaucracies for even a few of the moments they had left to live. I told her that to live like this, seeping blood into the gut, is to live with uncertainty – never knowing if the trickle might widen to a gush. Outside the patio doors, her grand-children had arrived in the garden. They were waiting to come in and see their grandmother. I wondered if we should stop and let them in, but she urged me to continue.

'But for some people, hospital is something they want to avoid so much that they're prepared to take the risk just in order to stay at home,' I went on. 'For some people, their priority is to be home with their family' – at this her husband at her side smiled, sympathetically – 'rather than be admitted again to a series of wards; they want to take their chances to live the life they most enjoy, for the weeks left to them.'

'What a stupid idea,' she said finally. 'What the fuck would someone do that for?' And I reached for the phone, and silently typed out the number for admissions.

That was the job, in the first weeks of the year, before the pandemic hit. It felt timeless, as if it hadn't changed much in a century, or had changed only in the specifics and not in the essentials, and wouldn't change for a century more at least. But I was wrong about that: there were only weeks left.

PRODROME

*'So the Plague defied all medicines; the very physicians were
seized with it, with their preservatives in their mouths ...'*
Daniel Defoe
A Journal of the Plague Year

The word 'prodrome' refers to that period in the course of a
viral illness when the virus first begins its work on the body
– the incubation period is passed, the sufferer begins to feel a
little unwell but is still able to function. The virus has not
begun its multiplication through the tissues of lung, skin, or
gut – those parts of the body most exposed to viral attack.
The word is Greek: *pro* means 'forward', and *dromos* can
mean running, a sally, an offensive. It's a term from military
history, co-opted to the lexis of medicine to describe that
moment in the course of the illness when an infection is
preparing its assault. The virus and the immune system
are running towards one another across the battlefield of
the body.

On 4 February I flew to New York to join a panel at the
city's Academy of Sciences and contribute to a discussion
about curiosity and wonder in science and medicine. United
Airlines had been sending me a hail of text messages and
emails for days, reminding me that if I'd been in China I
would be turned back at the US border. Despite sporadic
face masks among the travellers, the virus still seemed like

a faraway problem; although one that, increasingly, I found myself thinking about with a nagging sense of anxiety.

There's a masterful history of the 1918 Spanish Flu pandemic called *Pale Rider*, by Laura Spinney; a couple of years earlier I'd reviewed that book in a long essay for the *London Review of Books*, and a producer at Radio New Zealand had contacted me to ask if I'd do an interview about the piece, and also offer some perspectives on other pandemics. I thought about the Chinese travel ban and how the fear of the 'other' has long influenced how we describe diseases: in Madrid, 'Spanish' flu was known as the 'Naples Soldier'; the Senegalese called it 'Brazilian flu'; in Brazil it was 'German flu' – everyone had someone else to blame. The source of the 1918 pandemic is obscure, but of the three theories Spinney puts forward, the greatest likelihood tips towards an origin in China, it probably having arisen in communities where humans and poultry shared living and sleeping spaces.

The difference in time, logistics and other obligations all meant that this interview, via Skype, was the first thing I did when I reached New York. The absurd levels to which we're all now interconnected came home to me as I sat down, cross-legged and jet-lagged, in a New York hotel room to talk to a radio presenter seventeen hours into tomorrow. He asked me for predictions on how far the new coronavirus would spread. I remember saying that I had no crystal ball, but what I'd seen of infection control measures in China seemed impressive – I hoped very much it would be contained as SARS-CoV-1 had been contained, and that isolation measures in China would be effective. That day it was reported that 425 Chinese patients had died, and infection rates, for those who'd been tested, stood at just over 20,000.

*

The World Health Organization confirmed on 5 February that there was 'no known effective treatment' for the new coronavirus; despite the ban, US citizens were still being flown home from Wuhan and allowed in through American airports. I met my editors at the *New York Review of Books*, where we discussed Donald Trump, American hospital care, mental health, the lack of paid leave for either maternity or sickness in the US, and of course coronavirus. I'd not long written a piece for the magazine about the evolution of diagnostic categories in mental illness. In the field of psychiatry it has often felt as if where America leads, the rest of the world follows; no one I met in New York seemed to think that the same would be true for managing a public health crisis like coronavirus. No one was talking of emulating a 'US approach'.

The following evening the New York Academy of Sciences held the panel discussion, and on arrival I went to shake hands with the host, who was heavily pregnant. 'I can't,' she said, pulling her hand away, pointing it instead at her swollen belly. 'I can't afford to get sick.' I nodded and apologised, though I shook scores of other hands that night.

Flying out of Newark the next day I found myself in a departure terminal where every table was festooned with tablet computers on stalks. They flashed like gambling machines, entertainment as well as shopping opportunities. To speak to a companion it was necessary to peer over these screens. All food and all payment was to be ordered by touching the tablets. Maybe they wipe them clean regularly, I thought, as I watched a kid pick his nose then start playing with the screen. Waiting for my own flight I picked up the first email from my childrens' school about coronavirus, bundled in with information about mumps – something my colleagues and I were seeing more and more of in Edinburgh, as vaccination rates among the educated middle classes fell. There was, it insisted, no cause for concern, and anyone with symptoms who'd been in China was asked to stay away from school and contact their GP.

The same day it was reported that one of the doctors who had alerted the world media to China's coronavirus crisis, the ophthalmologist Li Wenliang, had died of it. The *Guardian* newspaper reported that 'Li was one of eight people authorities targeted for "sharing false information", in a heavy-handed approach that China's supreme court later criticised. He agreed not to discuss his concerns in public again. But in early January he treated a woman with glaucoma without realising she was also a coronavirus patient; he appears to have been infected during the operation.' The paper drew a parallel with Dr Carlo Urbani, an Italian doctor who worked in Vietnam for the WHO, and who in 2003 died of SARS-CoV-1 after recognising the threat the virus posed, and doing everything possible to halt its spread. On its website the WHO wrote of Urbani: 'because of his early detection of the disease, global surveillance was heightened and many new cases have been identified and isolated before they infected hospital staff'. Li didn't seem to have been given even that opportunity.

By the time I got home the threat was beginning to feel real: we were into the prodrome of the first wave and it was clear that the infection, having been silently, rapidly spreading across the country, was now ready to make its presence felt. More UK cases had been confirmed: one, a British businessman in Brighton who'd caught the disease in Singapore, was confirmed on 6 February – he was later linked to eleven other cases. That weekend was a grim milestone: the number of deaths in China surpassed those of the SARS-CoV-1 epidemic of 2002–3, at 811. The coronavirus of that particular outbreak was more dangerous by some measures: the 'case fatality rate' – the proportion of people who, having contracted the virus, subsequently died of it – was often higher than one in ten. And yet SARS-CoV-1 spread far more slowly than the new coronavirus, taking months instead of days to reach countries outside China. That slowness of spread, and its perilously high fatality rate, all helped to rein in SARS-CoV-1 – outbreaks were spotted quickly because a high proportion of those carrying it became very unwell. This new virus seemed to be transmitted more speedily; many people seemed to be carrying and spreading it without symptoms, making it much more difficult to isolate affected individuals and prevent them from passing it on.

Half term holidays followed: with my wife and three children I drove to Orkney, the archipelago of islands off the northern mainland of Scotland. I once worked as a GP in Stromness, in the west of mainland Orkney, and we have many friends there. After a few days' holiday my family went home and I took up a locum position as a GP on one of Orkney's outer islands for a week. There were no hospital facilities on the island and no X-ray machines – just a GP clinic with a wider than average selection of drugs, and the company of one of the island's nurses.

In the town of Kirkwall, on my way to the ferry, a message pinged from one of the NHS Orkney staff. Did I have time to drop by the hospital and be measured up for a 'face-fitting mask'? It disturbed me that the request came in such haste. Did they know something I didn't about the imminence of the outbreak? In Orkney? These masks, which are effective at blocking the droplets of coughs or sneezes that carry viruses, would never normally be needed by a GP, and only rarely by a hospital doctor. I had time if I dropped by the hospital right now, I replied, but had only an hour until my ferry was leaving for the outer isles. 'It won't be necessary,' came the reply, and it wasn't.

The ferry took a couple of hours; I arrived in darkness, buffeted by gusts of wind, met at the jetty by the outgoing GP who took me to one of the island's two pubs for some food. He handed me the pager, the keys to the surgery, then with relish ordered his first pint of beer in a while. The following day he left for a skiing holiday in Switzerland.

It was a week of storms – Ciara and Dennis – with the ferries mostly in harbour and the planes grounded. After I'd seen my morning patients there might be a couple of hours of light left to the day, which I'd spend walking on desolate, invigorating beaches, swords of wind chopping at the dunes and raising a miasma of sand that drifted around my ankles. I was free to explore the island, as long as I was never more than twenty minutes from the car in case of a call.

In the end, there were just three emergency calls in the course of my eight days on the island. Islanders' lives are governed by the weather, and the community appreciates that the price of living in such a beautiful part of the world is that access to hospitals and to specialist services can be fragile, and transfers delayed. A famous description by Jorge Luis Borges of the sea as 'violent and ancient, who gnaws at the foundations of the earth' comes to mind, when thinking about the way it can imprison this community, even as it protects it. I had to refer two patients for hospital tests – one for a heart problem, the other to rule out appendicitis. My having dosed them as best I could from the surgery's extensive pharmacy, they were able to cross to the mainland on the ferries that ran through the brief lulls in the gales.

Several people that week asked me about coronavirus, whether I'd seen any cases yet, whether I thought the news of it was exaggerated, but behind their questions was the unspoken anxiety of what such a virus would do if it got into an island such as theirs. It would very quickly overwhelm the healthcare capacity, the limited oxygen supply, the ability to transfer patients safely to hospital. Each morning I had been conducting a clinic in parallel with the island's nurses – for the first few days, Helen, and for the last few, Karen, both hugely experienced, extraordinary clinicians, with years of local knowledge of every islander and their difficulties. But with just one doctor and one nurse on the island, there was a brittle vulnerability to the provision of care that could seem unimaginable from the busy hospitals of the mainland. It lay beneath the surface of my everyday exchanges with the patients: usually unspoken, though we were all aware of it. I thought of the way that doctors in China had become seriously ill themselves, and how every year I pick up viruses and colds from patients that I have to shake off. This virus might not prove so obliging.

The Scottish Environment Protection Agency issued a flood alert across the archipelago, because of the height and ferocity of the waves. The wind was gusting over sixty miles per hour. When one of my patients needed to be flown off the island as an emergency that week, the atrocious weather made it a trial to arrange.

When I spoke to the hospital specialist in Aberdeen, she agreed with me that my patient needed to be seen urgently. Because of the storms, the air ambulances weren't flying. I explained that there were no routine air transfers, and no ferries; if the patient was going to get off the island it would need to be with the help of the Coastguard – the only organisation with boats and helicopters capable of travelling in these conditions. That it might be possible for me to persuade the Coastguard to take the patient by boat to Kirkwall, but the tests available there were limited, and there were no sub-specialists. There was a silence on the line as she took in this information, and then she said: 'Just do what you need to do to get the patient seen.'

The Coastguard were reluctant to commit the patient to a lifeboat in such storms, but in the end agreed to send a helicopter from Shetland.

I put off thinking about how I'd manage this kind of difficulty should coronavirus take hold in the island. At busy times Scotland's helicopter air ambulance service flies almost non-stop between urban centres and remote communities, taking patients to urgent medical care. The emerging protocols dictated that, as things stood, the helicopters would not be able to carry coronavirus patients. If someone on the island came down with it we were to order a dedicated ambulance over from Orkney's mainland, a journey of over two hours, and arrange transfer back again on the next scheduled ferry.*

Each island in Orkney has its own healthcare team: they are remote from one another geographically but their workloads are similar and they face similar challenges. They keep in contact through a weekly videoconference; the doctor or nurse on each island dials in to a central NHS server. That week I sat in the island clinic room with Karen as, one by one, clinicians from each of the other islands of the archipelago popped up on screen, boxed in their own livestream window. Over the videoconference we shared stories of the week's challenges, and offered one another peer to peer, island to island advice. There was a brooding anxiety over how we'd manage an outbreak; on many islands the clinicians come and go in shifts, and there was real concern that any healthcare worker might introduce the virus to the community

---

* These protocols have evolved since February 2020.

they were employed to help. One of the clinicians gave a virtual tutorial on multiple sclerosis – a particular problem of high latitudes – but the real value of the session was to make remote healthcare workers feel less alone.

News reports from Wuhan described a strict lockdown, efficiently policed, and I thought of all those densely packed apartments where people were becoming accustomed to exactly this kind of videoconferencing. We needed it to connect different islands in an archipelago, but there the technology was necessary to connect neighbours across a corridor.

Later, in Kirkwall, I managed to get my mask fitted. I was met in the hospital forecourt and led through three key-coded doors to reach a side room where a woman in burgundy scrubs and steel-framed glasses awaited me, having laid out some masks on a table. I could see five or six types, and she led me through them. 'These work better with women,' she said, 'and these ones if you've got a big jaw. But you'd better start with one of these.' She handed me a mask and asked me to put it on. It was a white cereal bowl of a thing, with blood-red elasticated straps. I made an idiotic hash of putting it on, at first upside down, and getting only one of the loops over my head. She had seen this many times before, and suppressed a smile. 'Ah, both straps over my head, then,' I said, turning it, and she nodded, letting the smile break out.

I suspected that from the moment we met on the hospital forecourt she had been sizing up my jaw and nose like a connoisseur: immediately the mask fitted perfectly, snugly to my cheeks. She gave a nod of satisfaction. 'I'm just going to put this over your head,' she said, and shook out a boxy polythene hood, silvered on four sides, with a hole in the one transparent side. I was cast back to primary school, it's Halloween, and I've a painted crate made up to look like a knight's helmet on my head; wearing a mask beneath the enclosing walls of the hood I began to feel the whispering edge of claustrophobia. The woman picked up a little spray bottle of liquid and poked it into an access hole in the front of the hood. 'This is Bitrex,' she said; 'it tastes *really* horrible. Just keep breathing through your mouth and tell me if you taste anything funny.' She began to scoosh and, my head now bathed in a fine mist of foul-tasting droplets, I took a few experimental breaths. 'It's the stuff they paint on kids' nails to stop them biting them,' she added. 'I think they used to put it in bleach once, too, so that kids spit it out.'

I remembered that stuff from a nail-biting childhood, but don't taste anything that brings those years back to me. 'Right, deeper breaths now, really fill your lungs'; I gulped obligingly. 'Now call out, loud as you like, 1, 2, 3, 4, 5, 6, 7, 8, 9, 10.' She led me through a few other hooded aerobics but, despite the extremest of contortions within the mask and hood, I couldn't taste anything at all, and finally I was authorised to get out of it. A taint of the Bitrex hung in the air, the faintest echo of those nail-biting years suspended in the atmosphere of this modern hospital wing in Orkney. I thought of the virus it was there to simulate: as tasteless and odourless as carbon monoxide and, to some, just as lethal.

Back in Edinburgh on 20 February I dropped into a schedule of work at my own GP practice, with occasional afternoon locums at the Edinburgh Access Practice, a clinic for the city's homeless population. I've worked in various incarnations of the Edinburgh Access Practice over the years, but at the moment it is temporarily housed in the basement of an old church at the west end of the city's Grassmarket. It's a church once dedicated to St Cuthbert, a medieval Northumbrian miracle worker who, said the Venerable Bede, 'saved the needy man from the hand of the stronger, and the poor and destitute from those who would oppress them'. The street it stands on is called Spittal Street, from the old name for 'hospital', and it lies along what was once the western boundary of the city. The defensive walls that stood there are long gone, but the traveller approaching from Glasgow would once have had to pass over the site of the clinic and through an arched gateway, its crown spiked with the heads of traitors and malefactors.

There are so many resonances of the word 'homeless', and as many ways of being homeless as there are people. There are the couch surfers and rough sleepers, precarious tenants and asylum seekers, the trafficked, rejected and ejected, ex-prisoners turfed out with nowhere to go, and the dreamers who've made harsh contact with reality – all of whom have found out to their cost that there is no room at the inn. The homeless have the worst health outcomes in our society – life expectancy for rough-sleeping men is just 46, and for women it's even worse, at 41. In the UK. By contrast, the lowest national average life expectancy globally is for the Central African Republic, where men average 52 and women 56.

The weather was still cold. I saw a woman who'd been trafficked from east Asia, who didn't speak any English and who was pregnant. For an hour I was passed between telephone interpreters, trying to find one that spoke a dialect close enough to her own. Eventually I was able to establish that the police were already involved, and was able to pass on information about how she might get more support. Two men just released from prison, needing prescriptions for the drugs to ease their anxiety – both housed in B&B accommodation. Written across the notes of one of them was the message 'DO NOT SEE THIS MAN ALONE'. Towards the end of the afternoon John, one of the practice nurses, called me through to take a look at someone's feet. He lay on the examination couch, his rolled-up trousers filthy, and on his sockless feet I could see the purple stains of frostbite flourishing across his toes. Many years ago I worked as an expedition doctor in polar regions, but I had never seen a case of frostbite as severe as his. It was shameful that it was contracted not in Siberia, or in arctic Canada, but right here, in my home city, on my own doorstep.

In Edinburgh things were changing fast; the weekend service asked if I could come by and be assessed there for a 'face-fitting mask', just as I'd been asked in Orkney, but I knew the size I'd need now anyway. Then the offer was rescinded: new guidance had appeared that said that for the kind of examinations I perform as a GP it would be enough to wear a less protective 'fluid-resistant' mask and follow the usual infection control procedures – aprons, gloves, eye protection. The 'face-fitting masks' were to be preserved for those performing the kind of procedures where you might be sprayed with saliva, or worse, such as intubations and endoscopies. The blizzard of correspondence through our email inboxes about issues of personal protective equipment felt surreal – in the course of my work as a GP people are always coughing in my face, and every winter I get ill with one virus or another. I always take the flu vaccine and, year on year, I muddle through without having to take a day off. The kind of protection being proposed was frighteningly robust, and made me conscious that this virus was something entirely new, posing a level of danger that I'd never in my career previously encountered.

Some GPs were finding the governmental advice infuriatingly inconsistent, but it was clear that tough decisions were having to be made with limited resources. As the virus ran towards us from all corners of the planet, time was running out. As GPs we were being urged to avoid suspected cases in case we spread it inadvertently to others. But for every confirmed case who'd been unwell enough to need testing or who had been tentatively diagnosed, there would perhaps have been many asymptomatic people who were spreading it around, and who'd never fit any of the criteria for being tested.* If testing was supposed to throw a cordon around affected individuals, it was a patchy and ineffective one at best.

By the third week of February Italy, Spain and France had all reported coronavirus cases, and on 21 February Lombardy reported its first cases resulting from spread within Italy, rather than among people who'd flown in with the virus – they still had only six confirmed cases. My wife's family is from Lombardy, not far from Pavia, and my mother- and father-in-law went into isolation. Italy reported its first deaths the following day, but several patients of mine were still relaxed enough about the virus to fly to Milan and travel from there to the Alps for skiing holidays.

Within four days Italy's reported cases went from 6 to 229 and China's approached 80,000. In the UK the total stood at 13, although amongst the other GPs I spoke to it seemed we had to assume that the virus was circulating at higher levels than were evident in the official figures. But China's were slowing while Italy's appeared to be gathering momentum: a new bulletin from the public health specialists at NHS Lothian asked me to tell anyone who'd been in Lombardy or Veneto within the last fourteen days, and who had symptoms, to self-isolate. 'First of all, for reassurance,' it added,

---

* It was later confirmed that the virus was circulating in Paris in December 2019.

'with regards Italy the area of concern is only for northern Italy – north of Pisa, Florence or Rimini.' I was not reassured.

I spoke that day with someone who was, in retrospect, my first Covid-19 patient: a man who'd just returned from Rome, but who had no symptoms other than feeling feverish with a very slight sore throat, and an irritating dryness in his chest – common enough symptoms for anyone just off a plane. According to the rules I'd been given he didn't have to isolate himself, and didn't justify getting tested because he hadn't been in northern Italy or in China. 'Have you got a thermometer?' I asked him, and toyed with the idea of dropping round to see if he had a fever. But then more calls and demands came through, and I didn't. The first case of Covid-19 caught within the UK rather than imported was confirmed three days later, on 28 February. That same day, the first death of a British citizen occurred, not caught within the UK, or in China, but aboard the *Diamond Princess* cruise ship moored off the coast of Japan.

INVASIVE PHASE

*'I must acknowledge that this time was terrible, that I
was sometimes at the end of all my resolutions, and that
I had not the courage that I had at the beginning.'*
Daniel Defoe
A Journal of the Plague Year

Strictly speaking viruses aren't 'alive' – they're brainless packets of genetic material wrapped in a fatty envelope, with proteins jutting from their surfaces. Those proteins are the skeleton keys with which viruses enter living cells; once inside, they hijack the cellular apparatus to manufacture copies of themselves. This process can go on until the cells burst, shedding more viruses and irritating the tissue they've infected. If that tissue is skin it may cause blistering (as happens with chickenpox or herpes); if the nose, lungs and windpipe, it may cause coughing and sneezing.

Whether they spread through the weeping fluid of blisters or through coughed airborne droplets, as far as viruses can be said to 'want' anything, they want the ability to fan out and take up residence in as many individuals as possible without limiting their spread through the death of their host. Effective viruses like influenza are, at any time, immensely broadly distributed among the population – it's estimated that between 10 and 20 per cent of people in the UK harbour influenza in the course of each year. They're endemic, meaning that we never truly get rid of them, but at the same time waves of newly evolved influenza strains pass seasonally around the world from year to year, as sections of the population become immune or partially immune to each one.

But viruses that cause illness in humans can also hide inside 'animal reservoirs', often without giving symptoms to the host animals, and the ability to do this increases the pool of distribution exponentially. These are called 'zoonotic' diseases, from the Greek *zōon*, meaning 'animal', and *nosos* meaning 'disease'. We humans share sixty-five infectious diseases with dogs, and comparable numbers of other infections with goats, pigs, horses, poultry, sheep and cows. Measles arrived via dogs or cows; influenza from pigs and ducks; tuberculosis from cows; the 'rhinovirus' of the common cold from horses. Most likely, zoonotic epidemics have been with us as a species for at least as long as we've kept animals, rather than hunted them.

At the weekend emergency centre in West Lothian, in the first week of March, it was evident just how thick the weekly traffic is between Italy and the UK. The skiing enthusiasts were all returning home, many with coughs and fevers. Cases of the virus were rising as quickly across society: we were now into a period equivalent to the 'invasive phase' of an infectious illness, when virus particles begin to proliferate exponentially within the body, producing observable symptoms. One among several calls: a man who'd flown in a day earlier, from the south of France, and who had a headache, exhaustion and a fever. According to the guidance I'd been given, he wasn't to be considered as a case of coronavirus – I informed him there was no official need for self-isolation. But the advice made me uneasy, and I asked him, if he could, to stay inside and off work for at least a week.

A family fresh from an Alpine holiday, with exhaustion and fevers; according to the location of their resort they were at risk, and they were referred to public health for testing. This was done by sending away an official form to public health – we GPs weren't told who turned out positive and who didn't.*

The computer system with which GPs read all medical records, make notes on each consultation and refer patients for specialist care, had new coronavirus codes added in early March. The idea was that anyone with Covid-19 registered in the system would be tagged with a special code that would keep track of the spread of the disease, as well as our Covid-19 workload as GPs. At this point, 'Advice given about 2019-nCoV' was the only code that I had plenty of opportunity to use.

Officially, we were still in the 'containment' phase of the outbreak, both in terms of the media messaging from government and in the communications GPs were receiving from public health authorities. That meant that we couldn't swab or check people ourselves for Covid-19, but that the authorities would 'test and trace' all suspected cases coming from disease hotspots, isolate them and thereby attempt to stop the spread through the general population. But with cases climbing so fast, in order to carry on with 'containment' of the virus it felt like we would need hundreds of call handlers to decide who should stay put, who should self-isolate and who should be tested. And hundreds more workers to trace every contact. Drive-through testing of people who'd been in affected areas was happening in Edinburgh, organised through the Regional Infectious Diseases Unit (RIDU).

---

* That didn't change until August, when a new system linked to national clinical records began to inform GPs of every coronavirus swab result.

By now fear was spreading, with some justification, and the situation was beginning to feel extremely serious. One of my patients, a taxi driver called Eddie, worked on a zero hours contract. He paid heavy fees to hire his vehicle, and handled the money of his passengers all day long. 'I can't afford to be off for two weeks,' he said. ' If I can't work for two weeks I'm bankrupt. Homeless, too, as I won't be able to pay my rent.'

As a doctor I'm accustomed to fielding my patients' concerns, to meeting anxieties with reassurances, but the way this outbreak was evolving, I felt powerless to soothe or placate anyone. One elderly lady requested a letter for her insurance company, to get her out of her package holiday; I explained that until the government changed its advice my letter wouldn't make any difference and she left, dejected. Another patient, a scientist who works in a lab with co-workers from all over the world, came into the clinic with a headache as if a mallet had dropped on his forehead, a fever of 39 degrees and a cough. He hadn't been in Italy, though his partner had recently returned from Bologna, and he had colleagues who'd been in China earlier in the year. I had to tell him that under the current rules, he hadn't been anywhere that meant I could get him tested.

I listened to his chest: it sounded as if he was developing a severe pneumonia, so I sent him to the hospital for a chest X-ray. The local hospital had started asking everyone with cough and fever attending for tests to wear a mask; 'but the radiographer wasn't wearing one,' my patient told me later, and though he isolated for a fortnight with his partner, she never showed any symptoms. In retrospect he almost certainly had Covid-19, but it was my first encounter with what an opaque and capricious virus it is, to affect people so variably, to leave everyone so uncertain as to whether they've had it or not.

The supected Covid cases began to increase among my patients, all with what we now recognise as classic symptoms, but none meeting the strict national criteria for getting tested. It seemed clear to me that the virus was out there in our communities: a plumber with cough and fever; a woman who had returned from Umrah in Saudia Arabia, vomiting with fever. And still we were being asked to arrange testing on people only if they'd arrived from Italy and east Asia. The media messaging on my daily news bulletins suggested the virus was still fairly contained, but with such poor access to diagnostic tests and so many calls about cough and fever, I had to assume that the situation was much worse than was being admitted.

Watching the news, I thought the measures Italy was taking seemed necessary, if extraordinary: field hospitals springing up, draconian lockdowns, rationing of access to ITU. I once studied with military medics for a Diploma in the Medical Care of Catastrophes, learning about building makeshift hospitals, about dividing clinics into 'clean' and 'dirty' zones, about planning urgent mass vaccination, about emergency medical supply chains. It felt surreal that those kinds of measures were now being discussed so close to home, in a country with a medical system at least as well equipped as our own – if not better.

On 5 March the UK recorded its first death, an elderly woman who had contracted the virus within the country. There was broadening public awareness of the gravity of the crisis, but at the same time, even as a doctor in receipt of all the public health bulletins, I was having trouble grasping the true scale of what was breaking over the country. On Saturday 7 March, the same day the UK reported more than 200 cases, I was out with friends, many of them doctors, jokes aplenty about nudging elbows instead of shaking hands. I stood in the corner of a pub packed for the rugby: England victorious over Wales. We went together to a sold-out concert in Edinburgh's Usher Hall – capacity 2,200 – crowds singing, people hugging, everyone pretending to forget about Covid-19 for a night. We knew it was around, we had all seen patients we suspected of the virus, and yet we felt fine – we theorised that perhaps it was less dangerous than the press were reporting, perhaps our medical work, and the routine bombardment by coronaviruses that it occasions, had offered us a measure of protection? I knew the virus was real, that it was spreading, but everyone I'd spoken to with symptoms seemed to be managing at home; a small voice at the back of my mind wondered – perhaps hoped – that some of the sources might be overreacting.

The following day, 8 March, the whole of the north of Italy was in lockdown, but Brits were still being allowed to fly home from there without quarantine. There were frightening stories from hospitals in Lombardy of insufficient ventilators, and operating rooms having to be used as intensive care units – even more frightening given that Lombardy was known to have a sophisticated network of hospitals, and more than double the ITU beds available, per head of population, than are generally maintained in the UK.

My brother-in-law was scheduled to move home to Lombardy from southern Spain that week, and had packed all his possessions into the back of a van, intending to manage the drive over two or three days. But with the worsening spread of the virus he realised he might not be allowed to drive over the border, and would have to go by public transport. He spent 8 March storing his possessions in his landlady's cellar, to be collected when all this might be over, then took a train across Spain from Córdoba to Barcelona. People there were still thick in the streets, he said, kissing and holding hands as he walked among them in mask and gloves. He took another train from Barcelona to Marseille, where he waited in a corner of the station, keeping himself as far from others as he could. In Nice he met other Italians in masks and gloves, racing to get home, many to look after family members. They were mocked by local kids for their masks and gloves, and name-called *'Chinoise'*.

The Italian border was closed – shocking after all these years of Schengen Area borders in Europe – but he had only to show his Italian ID card, fill in a declaration of why he was travelling into Italy, that he had family there, and that he understood the situation, and he was allowed to continue.

It took him two trains to reach Genova from the border, where the police were uncharacteristically helpful and attentive; the atmosphere was one of gentle camaraderie, he said, and grim obstinacy in the face of the crisis. From Genova he took an (empty) local train home to his village. He'd spend fourteen days in the basement of his parents' house, avoiding all contact with them until he was sure he didn't have the virus.

By 9 March swathes of Italy's north were 'Category 1', meaning that anyone who had passed through them was to self-isolate for fourteen days, even if they didn't have any symptoms. An American journalist reporting from Lombardy flew back into JFK airport in New York, tweeting her surprise at being allowed to walk freely through arrivals with no one querying where she had been, or whether she had a fever. In the UK, newspapers were full of the absurdity of the supposed 'quarantine' in Italy, given that people were given free passage out of the country.

The epidemiologist Max Roser began publishing graphs online showing the benefit of doing all that you can to slow the spread of a virus, even if it was inevitable that it would reach everyone eventually. He showed two curves – one with no limits on how the virus might be allowed to spread through a population which looked like a Himalayan arête, and another with extreme 'social distancing' measures that looked more like the gentle swell of the South Downs. The same number of people would be affected in both, but the second had a much slower ascent to the peak and a slower come down, meaning the health services wouldn't be over-whelmed by the peak.

The following day 'Category 1' was extended to cover the whole of Italy. There were riots in the prisons, as prisoners protested about visits being stopped, frightened of being left to die, abandoned by a depleted prison staff. Stories emerged of care homes in Italy being deserted by their staff because of the virus, of the military coming in to find residents dead in their beds.

In Edinburgh we GPs had an email from the Regional Infectious Diseases Unit pleading with us not to call them for advice. The volume of calls from anxious GPs passing on the concerns of travellers to and from disease hotspots around the globe was making the on-call system untenable.

There was another message detailing how Scotland would approach the management of people unwell with Covid-19 in the Highlands and Islands; how we might transfer people off islands to the units in Aberdeen or Inverness, in isolation. Reading it felt surreal, and to me it seemed unworkable; I wondered how many involved in creating the protocol had ever been involved with an island transfer: the enforced proximity waiting for ferries or flights for hours on end;

the logistical difficulties caused by weather; the speed with which an island's medical resources are overwhelmed. Six or seven people are required to come together just to make an air strip safe for a helicopter or plane to land. Meanwhile, in Italy they were having to treat the sick in hospital corridors.

I woke up on 10 March to a WhatsApp message from a colleague – though we'd seen plenty of suspected cases already at our own practice, the first few Covid-19 cases from our patch of Edinburgh had been officially confirmed with testing, all people returning from Italy. They had a fever, a forehead headache and a dry cough. We were all waiting for the news, but it still came like a cold slap. Everything about the way we worked would have to change. Planes were still flying in from Italy and France. Websites were telling worried people to phone their GP, while each morning we GPs were picking through emails to find out what had changed. Protective suits were to be saved for hospital staff and paramedics at the bedsides of sick people shedding the virus. I began to wake more often at night, anxiously re-running conversations with patients I had had during the day: wondering if I had done the right thing in telling someone to stay at home, or not; wondering how my clinic would manage to go on caring for its patients if the staff began to succumb.

At the surgery, we decided to slash the number of appointments offered by 50 per cent, filled the new space with phone appointments, and used a new code in the medical records: 'Telephone triage due to Covid-19 restrictions.' All the same, a colleague and I still made five visits that day to frail, elderly, housebound patients – among the most lonely, isolated people in our community, all of them over eighty-five, and all asking anxiously about the virus, trying with their questions to gauge our own levels of concern.

There were plenty of nervous jokes among my patients that day about the coming Coronageddon, but only one who phoned in with the now familiar dry cough, drenched in sweat and a fever of 39 degrees. He lived alone, hadn't been abroad for months, and I told him to stay home for a week at least and have friends drop off food at his doorstep – I'd ring in a week to see how he was, and asked him to let me know if his breathlessness worsened. Pubs were still open, and that evening my GP colleagues and I had a meeting in one that felt like a boozy council of war, sharing stories we'd heard of patients in hospital with the virus, and ideas for how to protect the practice, should we each catch it. I remembered planning meetings for the 'swine flu' of 2009, but they were nothing like this, and the threat felt nowhere near as real.

Only two and a half weeks after Italy's first cases were reported, the WHO called Covid-19 a pandemic. The speed at which this virus was moving was unprecedented. The UK Budget was delivered and the NHS was told it would have whatever it needed. I had my doubts. The numbers of deaths in China continued to drop – just 19 new infections. By then they'd reported almost 81,000 cases and just over 3,000 deaths.

At the school gate one of the other parents, a consultant physician, told me that the flimsy masks and aprons we were being advised to use in assessing Covid patients were all we were going to get – not gowns as recommended by the WHO. 'They're safe enough if you wash your forearms afterwards,' she said. A helpful message signed by senior members of all the government health departments, health boards, Royal Colleges and the General Medical Council (GMC) came on 11 March: it said that I'd be expected, in the coming weeks, to go beyond what I'm accustomed to dealing with, but that

I can be reassured that the GMC and health board would support me and my decisions through the crisis. 'Clinicians may need to depart, possibly significantly, from established procedures in order to care for patients in the highly challenging but time-bound circumstances of the peak of an epidemic.' It felt good to me that the GMC was at my back, rather than on my back, for a change.

Ireland closed its schools and universities on 12 March, and the United States precipitously blocked arrivals from European countries within the Schengen Area – planes, it seems, were still flying, but only US citizens would be allowed into the country on arrival. My patients' attitudes to the virus that day were an odd mixture of terrified and laissez-faire: a grandmother who had taken on the care of her three grandchildren worried over her ability to go on caring for them should the virus reach her and her husband. A man with advanced cancer, spread to the liver, thought everyone was overreacting. A mother of a 7-year-old girl who was home with fever and cough asked whether that meant she should also be self-isolating.

To those who had mild symptoms – headache, or a dry cough – the official answer was always the same: as long as they hadn't travelled to a recognised global hotspot of disease, then I couldn't get them tested for Covid-19, and I didn't need to inform them to self-isolate. Not yet, not yet, was the refrain – the government and the health board and the Chief Medical Officer were still sending me daily updates and, as far as they were concerned, we were still in the first of the four phases of a pandemic: 'containment'. But it felt wrong – with the virus now so obviously highly contagious between individuals, and surviving on surfaces for several hours, any one of my patients might have it. It was a relief when that day we switched to the next phase of 'delay', where we might accept that anyone with symptoms could have the virus, no matter where they had travelled, and the only thing to do to keep yourself well was to avoid crowded places, wash your hands, don't touch your face and, if at all possible, stay away from work.

That's not an option for GPs, of course – that day my practice moved to a system whereby we stopped bringing people into the clinic at all if we could help it, and dealt with as many queries over the phone as possible, shunting those less urgent concerns into some imaginary locus in the future when everything might start to go back to normal. Over morning coffee, a colleague and I joked about getting a HazMat suit each, and moving directly to visiting only the most seriously ill in their homes while hermetically sealed in our own isolation units. We joked, but knew it could be coming.

I spent the afternoon doing a men's clinic for the city's rough sleepers and those with no fixed address, some of whom sleep in Bethany Trust dormitories, 'night shelters' that ordinarily run through winter and as late into the year as Easter. In my morning surgery in a leafier part of the city *every patient* had asked me about the virus. My homeless patients had, it seems, more pressing concerns. About half went to shake my hand, and thought me cowardly for bumping elbows instead. For the most part, people without homes or income, who live on the margins of society, whose concerns are so much more immediate, saw this as something for others to worry about – something for the kind of people who go on flights and cruises. Homeless people living in shelters and in temporary accommodation, couch-surfing around the city wherever they could find a place to sleep, were undoubtedly at higher risk than the general population. But it was clear, too, that they faced so many obstacles just to get through each day that the virus was either too intangible to take seriously, or perhaps they simply had less to lose.

By the time I emerged from the clinic the UK Prime Minister Boris Johnson had told *everyone* with cough and cold symptoms to stay home for a week. At last! I thought. GPs were again told that more protective equipment was coming, but the droplet-resistant masks still wouldn't be available. Everyone with a beard who worked in a high-risk environment of Covid-19 patients had been asked to shave it off, as the masks don't work if there's hair between them and the skin. Anyone with religious or cultural objections was to speak with their line manager.

The relentless news cycle of what was happening in Europe and the rest of the world was strangely enthralling, grimly addictive: it satisfied something of our human fascination with fear, and pandered to our wish to seek examples of what we might one day have to deal with ourselves. A friend told me she watched compulsively in an attempt to foresee what was coming to us, but also because this pandemic was uniting us as human beings across borders and cultures. It didn't matter whether you're in Iran, where video footage showed rows of body bags being hurled into mass graves, or Rwanda, where everyone getting on a bus had to publicly wash their hands before embarking, or Bulgaria, where they'd just had their first deaths, we were all at risk, and we'd all get the virus the same way – through an infected human contact. But despite the horror of the images from Iran, the footage coming out of Italy was still more likely what we'd face in the UK – hospital corridors stacked with beds, problems with oxygen supply, lack of sufficient ventilators for our ageing population.

*

Friday the Thirteenth, and there was an atmosphere of dread in our morning meeting at the news from Italy: there weren't enough ventilators to go round, or nurses; people were being buried without funerals. The practice WhatsApp group was renamed 'Dream Team CoronaCombat' in an attempt at levity. There was an air of quiet resignation at what was coming, but an edge of bunker humour, too. One of the clinic thermometers broke, and I went online to buy another – £30 versions were changing hands for £125. But virologists were learning about Covid-19 all the time and, for all their horrors, the Chinese and Italian experiences meant that we were better prepared than we might have been.

One of my patients that day was Mr Mirandola, an Italian gentleman in his late eighties. He told me that the virus was Mother Nature getting back at us. 'Too many people!' he said, and chuckled. 'All us oldies need clearing out!' I didn't share his glee. The lab had stopped accepting viral swabs from GPs in order to scale up their testing capacity for the virus for hospital inpatients and, unless someone was admitted to hospital, they didn't get a test.

It was on 13 March that the first death in Scotland was announced, in Edinburgh. One of my own patients was a close contact of the victim but wasn't herself swabbed – she was just told to stay home for fourteen days with her husband and children. Another family – husband, wife, two children – phoned me to report a new cough and I told them that they'd need to stay in for a fortnight and arrange deliveries of food. They were incredulous: 'This isn't the middle ages,' the dad said to me. 'Surely they've got ways to treat this.'

The following day, Saturday 14 March, Spain would follow Italy into lockdown, with planes turning back halfway. The UK policy of allowing schools to stay open came under attack. It was obvious we needed new ways to slow the spread, particularly among the over-65s. One of my colleagues purchased us HazMat suits from eBay for home visiting, just in case; in the space of days, what had seemed like a surreal joke became reality.

That weekend I spent some time on the phone to an elderly woman living with her husband who has dementia. They were already barely coping at home despite carers coming in throughout the day and weekly visits from me. But when any GP might be carrying the virus asymptomatically, trying to assess their problems face to face felt like a luxury we couldn't afford – we had to reduce home visiting to a minimum, almost to life-or-death situations. So the old lady and I had a difficult conversation about limiting those visits, and she had some weighty decisions to make about her own priorities. Both she and her husband were living on a tightrope of frailty, perpetually on the verge of admission to hospital, which no longer seemed like a safe space to be, and now she had to decide how much risk she was prepared to live with at home. It was clear that managing Covid-19 was going to be about so much more than treating surges of people unwell with the virus – it was going to be about transforming the way we could practise medicine.

A young man called me to say that a Belgian tourist had collapsed in his workplace five days ago. He'd spent two hours with the Belgian man and his daughters, while waiting for ambulance paramedics to come. Those daughters came by the workplace to inform them all that it had been confirmed the collapsed man had the virus. No one had contacted the workplace to tell the staff they'd all been exposed, and the victim's daughters were walking around in Edinburgh *not* isolated, despite the near certainty of their own infection.

These were the kinds of stories that governments had been hearing but the public had not, forcing the policy to shift from 'containment' of the virus to 'delay'. The public health authorities had a good idea how many people out there were already coughing and spreading it; they knew that the time for containment had long passed.

I phoned the public health authorities and they confirmed the case – no, they hadn't traced his contacts as far as the workplace of my own patient, but yes, they would now include it in the follow-up. It felt like we had already lost the fight to contain Covid-19, and it was only a matter of time until the practice staff themselves began to get ill.

Of the thirteen coronavirus emails I had to read that morning of Friday 13 March, before starting to manage my own patients, this was the most relevant:

Subject: COVID 19 complete change in UK policy: please read now
Importance: High
Dear Colleagues
The UK coronavirus policy completely changed late last night.

We will not be testing people who have mild symptoms. People with mild symptoms are advised to stay at home for 7 days, that they will not be tested and that they do not need to seek healthcare (even by phone).

Patients with mild symptoms who have been referred to the testing service but have not yet been tested or do not have an appointment already (mainly today) will not be tested. Please advise your patients of this and recommend they stay at home for 7 days from onset of symptoms.

The guidance on specified countries we have been using up til now has been completely rescinded.

We will advise as soon as possible on guidance for the elderly, people with immunocompromise, pregnant and children. We are in a state of flux just now.

Further guidance is to follow re healthcare workers in practices.

NHS inform has not yet been updated. It will no doubt catch up in due course.

For patients with symptoms requiring admission to hospital please organise admission in the usual way, noting the presenting symptoms.

Thank you

If testing of suspected cases was being abandoned, I realised with a strange mixture of terror and relief that the government must be moving towards a 'herd immunity' strategy. Relief because it made the difficult work of contact tracing redundant, but terror because slowing the virus, but continuing to allow it to spread through the community, could lead to horrifying numbers of deaths. The city's universities were closing down, and that afternoon our Personal Protective Equipment (PPE) allocations arrived at a depot. Each bundle was supposed to be delivered to the appropriate GP practice after the weekend, but there was a scramble for it, and a rumour was already spreading that there was none left – that practices who didn't send a representative to the depot that afternoon would be left with none.

My parents, both in their seventies, called and asked me whether this was all as serious as it sounded. 'Yes,' I told them, 'stay home. I'll get your shopping.'

I started reading Boccaccio's *Decameron*, the Italian classic narrated from a fourteenth-century Florentine villa by ten aristocrats, all in lockdown from the plague. Over ten days, each of the ten tells a story to help pass the time – making a hundred tales. Boccaccio borrowed most of his stories from other sources – many were old classic tales in their own right before he stole or borrowed them for his book, and I flicked through them restlessly. Stories of lewd nuns, double-crossed simpletons and duplicitous priests weren't going to be helpful in getting me through the next few weeks. I was still thinking in terms of weeks for how long it would take to bring this virus under control, rather than months or years. I had more luck with Daniel Defoe's *A Journal of the Plague Year*, a semi-fictional account of life in London through the plague of 1665, that Defoe is thought to have based on the diaries of his uncle, Henry Foe (Defoe was only five years old in 1665). Passage after passage could have been written about our own modern-day 'plague', and I underlined many of them, as if they had something to teach me not just about surviving epidemics, but about the timelessness of human experience in the face of infection.

Four days later, on Tuesday 17 March, the practice felt oddly quiet – people were stunned by the implications of the guid-ance delivered by the Prime Minister the night before, to avoid going out, to avoid restaurants and theatres, to self-isolate for fourteen days if anyone in the household has symptoms. Exceptional, necessary, belated advice. Of the twenty people I spoke to on the phone, a couple certainly had the virus – a new headache, fever, cough, malaise and exhaustion. I coded them 'suspected coronavirus infection' and gave them advice to stay in with their whole families, and call us if they got worsening breathlessness, before add-ing them to a lengthening 'to do' list to remind me to check in on them. As healthcare workers we'd been told to follow the same advice as everyone else – stay off work for fourteen days if anyone at home had a cough or fever; adjacent practices to my own were already losing staff, and we were clamouring for testing. Hospital clinics were being cancelled wherever possible, all elective surgery postponed. It felt as if we were clearing the decks for an onslaught the likes of which hadn't been seen in over a century. The government's brief flirtation with a policy of herd immunity appeared to be over, and a net was closing in on the whole of society – I could feel a UK-wide lockdown coming, and soon. Every day I was speaking with families stressed at being ordered to confine themselves together in their homes because of the symptoms of one family member; I wondered if they'd feel more able to cope once *everyone* in the community was ordered to stay home.

On Wednesday 18 March we heard that UK schools would be closing, too, and my wife and I – like millions of parents – would be contending with the competing needs of our three kids, the virus, her work and the NHS. We took the children to the local library the day before it closed, and stamped out stacks of books and story CDs – I realised it could be months before it opened again.

My wife contacted her GP in Lombardy; the situation is, he said, very grave, and he wished us luck with what is to come. Several of his colleagues in neighbouring villages had died through seeing infected patients. Many priests had died, too – shocking but not surprising, given how many of them shake rows of hands outside churches, and offer communion into the open mouths of their congregations. I messaged a medical contact in Beijing, the Chinese translator of my books, the surgeon Dr Xiangtao Ma, who said things were improving there, with few new cases. 'As you know, isolation is the only effective method to stop the virus,' he added, and asked that I give thought to the mental health of my patients as much as to their physical needs. He ended on a sanguine note: 'People will have to change their habits for a while. The spring is coming.'

The masks we'd had delivered from NHS central stores were originally stamped with an expiry date of July 2016, perhaps warehoused for the swine flu epidemic of 2009, but someone had affixed new stickers stamped August 2021. It didn't bother me – what can expire about a mask? – but some people must have written to the government in horror. An email came from Gregor Smith, then the Deputy Chief Medical Officer for Scotland: 'I would like to clarify that this stock has been subject to rigorous assessment and shelf-life extension by the manufacturer and is therefore safe to use. I hope this allays any concerns you may have.' It was obvious that what pandemic preparations had been in place had slipped.

My 'clinic' was almost all on the phone, and I had finished by 5 p.m. I had an hour to spare before an evening shift performing 'telephone triage' for the evening and weekend service – ringing anyone concerned about their symptoms and gauging who needed to be seen in hospital. I walked slowly through the city towards the clinic base, past all the closed bars and cafés, wondering if I'd have to turn up to work hungry. The first restaurant I passed, Encounter China, was closed but an Italian place, Cafe Artista, was still open for a plate of spaghetti – although the owner told me he'd close the following day.

A colleague sent me a copy of the research study from Imperial College that had changed government policy into one of lockdown, or 'suppression' of the virus, rather than a 'mitigation' policy whereby it's assumed that the bulk of the population would have to catch and develop herd immunity to the virus. The latter strategy would need vulnerable, elderly or particularly susceptible people to hide or 'shield' from the virus while it's in general circulation, which might take months or even years. It was the first time I had heard the term.

The paper estimated just how dangerous this disease would be without active suppression and distancing. Just 'mitigation', with minor changes to how society functions, would, the paper's authors thought, lead to hundreds of thousands of deaths. With full societal lockdown they hoped to limit the deaths to the tens of thousands.

Edinburgh's medical centre for telephone triage is on the south side of the city, in an old convalescent hospital built after the First World War. For my shift that evening there were ten or twelve of us – GPs, district nurses and telephonists – all in an open plan office on the ground floor of the old building. We passed around a single packet of antiseptic wipes with which to clean each workspace before starting. The wipes might have been in short supply, but there was a cupboard stuffed with chocolate bars and packets of crisps. 'This is the best base,' said one of my colleagues, holding out a tin for my 25 p donation, 'it has a tuckshop with 1980s prices.' I spent the evening with a recently glued and Sellotaped headset, one finger in my uncovered ear, phoning patient after patient with the same symptoms – dry irritating cough, headache, chest feeling tight, some rib pain – giving advice and arranging for the sickest, who might need oxygen, to be seen at one of the hospital bases.

One of the district nurses on duty was Christine, a

Highlander who on day duty works my patch of the city. Her quiet competence, and accent down the phone line of English lilted with Gaelic, always comes as a relief to the ear. We joked about the tuck shop, swapped stories of shared patients, but when a call came in for a visit the atmosphere shifted. With a colleague she suited up in mask, visor and overalls, and gave a grim smile and a wave. 'Wish us luck!' she said. None of us were accustomed, yet, to having these barriers of plastic between us and our patients.

As GPs we're taught to value the subtleties of human communication – to glean as much from what the patient *doesn't* say as from what they do say. As trainees we have to submit videos of our consultations to demonstrate how carefully we attend to body language, to silences, to the way patients hold or evade eye contact. At this stage of the pandemic we were consulting for the most part on the phone, and for me those encounters felt alien, and profoundly unsatisfying. In happier days there was a sense of fellowship to my meetings with patients; on a crackling phone line, I could barely make myself understood to the anxious, ill person on the other end. Carrying out home visits in a mask, I feel like a surgeon looming over someone on the brink of anaesthetic oblivion.

'Social distancing' measures should of course have come in earlier, to buy us time – we all saw that then. We'd been like toddlers on the beach, fascinated by the waves edging ever closer up the sand, but who still squeal with shock when the water rolls over our toes. None of us could be persuaded to jump back until the disease was already on us.

That weekend supermarkets and Amazon dropped selling books, as they were considered dispensable items; warehouse workers needed to be shifting food and toilet rolls instead. I stopped off at the local bakery on the way to work to buy cake for all the practice staff, correctly guessing that by the following day it would be closed. So many more cases of cough and fever on the phone, but more than that, we were now struggling to address a mental health crisis with the feeble but essential minimum of telephone calls. I spoke to several people facing bankruptcy, many with panic attacks, who couldn't sleep.

Our practice building has only one entrance, and there was no way to make a 'green' or a 'red' area for separating Covid patients from others. To make the best of it we opted to use our now-empty waiting room as a Covid clinic, laid out a mop and a bucket of disinfectant, and bought a folding clinic screen on the internet to offer a minimum of privacy. The virus could hang in droplets in the air, we were told, so a larger space would make the air less dangerous to breathe, and we opened the window. Patients would wear masks, and anyone with throat problems I'd see outside, where I hoped the perpetual Edinburgh breeze might carry viral particles away from their gaping mouths before they could settle on me. New IT services in the NHS usually take months, but a system for video calls with patients was implemented in the space of a few days. From my computer I could send a link to a patient's smartphone which would patch them through to the computer in my office. I used it to diagnose a child's rash on a screen, and with a woman in lockdown suffering chest pains, not from the virus but from rising panic.

One of the patients I spoke with asked, 'Isn't this all a bit much, Dr Francis? I mean, it's hardly bubonic plague!' I agreed to a point, but asked if she'd watched the news from abroad. The plague may have killed around a quarter of the population with each epidemic, while Covid-19 seemed to be killing 'only' around 2 per cent. But at the same time, outbreaks of plague are easier to spot, and consequently control. With the power of this coronavirus to be transmitted without symptoms, kill 10–15 per cent of the most fragile people in our communities, make a much larger proportion very ill, and with its long-term effects still unknown, I asked her if she might prefer we do nothing.

In a bid to contain the spread of infection through GP clinics, 'Covid clinics' or 'Hot Hubs' were planned to go live the following week: it made sense to concentrate all the suspected cases in one place rather than have patients coughing the virus over the surfaces of every GP surgery in the country. At first it was presumed these hubs would have access to better PPE than us out in the community, but no – they were to have the same disposable aprons and surgeons' masks as the rest of us.

Outside, there were still too many people on the streets, and one of the London hospitals had called a critical incident. On the news there was talk of Italy needing a European Central Bank bailout, and of Spain urgently seeking to 'flatten its curve' within a fortnight. By 21 March, the spring equinox, thirteen doctors in Italy were dead of the virus. Three months earlier my wife and I had thrown a party to celebrate the winter solstice, with friends and neighbours crushing into our house and garden. We'd planned to hold another party at the spring equinox, but the people squeezed together in the rooms of our house, the hugs and chinking glasses, already seemed to belong to another age.

Barra in Scotland's Outer Hebrides closed, the island literally self-isolating to keep its community safe. Kate Forbes, the Scottish finance secretary and Member of the Scottish Parliament for Skye & Lochaber, asked people *not* to take to the Highlands and Islands in their campervans. As I had seen in Orkney, the isolation of remote communities both protected them and threatened them: remoteness from urban centres meant remoteness from medical infrastructure and resources. Any small jump in Covid cases could swamp a small community. During the Spanish flu pandemic, remote communities endured some of the highest mortality rates: in Tonga, the mortality rate was 10 per cent, in Samoa, 20 per cent. There were some Inuit communities of Alaska where 50 per cent of the people died.

Driving down the motorway to a shift in the out of hours centre that weekend, I saw that the traffic signs ordinarily dedicated to accidents, deviations and seat-belt admonitions had all switched to public health: 'COVID-19 –ESSENTIAL TRAVEL ONLY.' They were a forewarning of the Prime Minister's announcement, on Monday 23 March, that everyone must now stay home, and that there were just four permitted reasons for leaving the house: essential work; to buy food; to exercise once daily; or to care for someone. Everyone was in lockdown whether they were ill or not. It seemed incredible that we'd come to such measures in such a short space of time, but I was grateful that I no longer had to make the nerve-wracking decisions about whether to advise people to stay in or allow them to go out. In just three days a further three Italian doctors had been reported dead of Covid.

The day after lockdown was announced I pedalled to my clinic, exchanging guilty looks with everyone else who was out, as if we were all preparing our 'essential worker' alibis. Roadworks were still going on, and builders were labouring at a couple of house extensions I passed. I thought how much the crisis had triggered the wholesale recalibration of the prestige of different jobs: shelf-stacker, refuse-collector, care-provider, all seen for their value and essential utility.

Doctors and nurses, too, of course, but we already enjoyed a measure of prestige (though surveys consistently show that doctors aren't the most trusted professionals – nurses are). On my return journey the roadworkers and builders had disappeared.

The ITU of the city's Royal Infirmary was operating at 20 per cent capacity; a friend who worked there said it was as if they were waiting for a deluge. GPs were sent guidelines about how to assess levels of 'respiratory distress' without coming close to a patient, just by watching breathing movements and measuring oxygen levels of the blood. A method of gauging oxygen content of the blood over the telephone just by asking the patient to count as long as they could in one breath, the Roth method, was widely disseminated to GPs, then rapidly discredited after it was shown to be tragically inaccurate in cases of Covid-19 pneumonia.

The Covid patients I spoke with that day included an agoraphobic woman who picked up the virus at her aunt's funeral. She had the headache that's so characteristic of the infection, the dry cough that she couldn't suppress for more than a few words, and was feeling acutely breathless in the mornings – though her sense of gasping for oxygen seemed to fade over the course of the day and she felt well overnight. We discussed how, after years of agoraphobia and anxiety, paradoxically she was feeling better now that no one else was allowed out. She had taken herself off all her anxiety medication for the first time in years. Other anxious patients of mine, habitual worriers, reported a similar sense of relief: the worst actually *had* happened, and that realisation brought an unexpected sense of liberation.

That week the Italian cases began to drop for the first time, while in the US cases were burgeoning. The WHO chief described how the first 100,000 cases took a month to be confirmed, the next 100,000 cases just eleven days, and the third 100,000 cases took only four days. Very soon we'd be talking in terms of millions of cases.

The Health Secretary wrote to tell me that Covid hubs would mean I'd shortly be able to get back to my usual workload. That email was quickly followed by another from NHS Lothian telling me of the 'desperate' need for more volunteers – could I put more of my usual work aside? The hub had just opened and I'd signed up for Thursdays and Sundays, but there was little slack available now that the schools were all closed, and when not in my own clinic I'd be at home with my children. Many of my colleagues were reluctant to sign up because work in the hubs was considered 'ad hoc', and offered no sickness pay if you caught Covid while working at them; there were similarly no 'in harness' benefits for the families of anyone who died of it. At the same time, we GPs were trying to support our own patients: if the network of general practice collapsed, it was obvious that hospitals would struggle to cope.

It was a weary week, the first week of UK lockdown, oppressive with the weight of all the misery this pandemic had unleashed. We'd been told so often in the last few years that mental health is the equal of physical health in terms of the respect and attention it should be accorded. But suddenly mental health was being obliged to take second place in order to protect the physical health of the community's most vulnerable members. One day, 25 March, almost everything I dealt with related to mental health – all those people cooped up at home, watching their debts accumulate while their prospects dwindled, as vast swathes of the economy devoted to leisure, travel and tourism collapsed. There was so much regret out there, stewing in isolation – people wishing they'd seen this coming and changed their work or their finances to prepare.

One of the many problems general practice was facing was a surge in patients with chronic mental health problems such as schizophrenia being discharged from long-term hospital stay. It was assumed they would be safer outside an institution, and from the point of view of Covid risk that was true – but these were all people whose mental health was so precarious and volatile that they were thought to need hospital care to be safe. I was asked if I'd take over the care of one long-term patient with schizophrenia, including her regular injections of antipsychotics, and was told she *would* turn up for her injections, because if not she'd be breaking her 'community treatment order'.

There was the misery, too, of people for whom home was no refuge, obliged to shut themselves in with aggressive or violent partners. The foster carers of troubled kids. The couples in immiserating marriages. The single parents barely coping. Every week I spoke with people in all those categories and more, while fielding a huge number of calls about who could be considered resilient enough against the virus to continue attending their 'essential' work, and which essential workers now had to stay at home. And all the while, the economy was buckling, shrieking, twisting into a wall of coronavirus.

In London the ExCeL Centre was being turned into a 4,000-bed hospital, and New York's governor was screaming for 30,000 ventilators. India was attempting a lockdown of 1.3 billion people.

My friend Polly teaches in China, but had been sent back early in the Wuhan outbreak to the UK. Now she flew back to take up her job again in Shanghai – China had done so well in bringing its epidemic under control. The flight was almost full, but all the other passengers with her were in suits and masks. A day later, all visas and flights were cancelled. Every worker at the airport in Shanghai had full PPE with suits and masks, she told me – better than the PPE issued to doctors and carers in the UK. She went directly from the airport to a testing centre in a sports hall, where everyone on the plane was tested. They waited together there for the result – six hours, as compared to the three or four days it was taking for us in Scotland to get results – and because she tested negative she was allowed home (anyone testing positive was transferred to a government quarantine facility, along with all those passengers who had been seated nearby). Nevertheless, a device was fitted to her door to enforce a fourteen-day quarantine, and she was visited twice daily by a doctor to check her temperature. 'My compound was very supportive,' she told me. 'They allowed me to have deliveries which they brought themselves via the security guards in suits, and they took my rubbish out for me every day.' It felt as if China would solve the problem of the virus long before Europe would, but at the cost of a degree of state intrusion into the private lives of citizens that few Europeans would wish to contemplate.

Every NHS service was being stopped or scaled back. Cancer screening, new stroke clinics, IVF, sexual health (though with social distancing, STI transmission was plummeting). ECGs and X-rays were to be reserved only for the critically ill, or those in whom cancer was suspected.

Prince Charles tested positive, with 'mild symptoms', and was recuperating at Balmoral, though the nation had just been told not to stress the fragile resources of rural communities by travelling to the Highlands. There was mention of taking over the Scottish Exhibition Centre in Glasgow to make a giant Covid hospital, but I wondered if Balmoral might not be a better choice. Good views, fresh Highland air, plenty of bedrooms, relative isolation.

By the final weekend of March the virus wasn't slowing in Italy, which was recording over 900 deaths a day, or in Spain, and was accelerating in New York. A German finance minister committed suicide. I watched maps online showing the number of cases as red dots blooming into wide circles, like spores in a petri dish. In just a week the number of deaths doubled, from 13,000 globally to 27,000 – the swine flu of 2009 saw about 20,000 confirmed deaths worldwide. Epidemiological studies were published showing the virus has the potential to cause 30 million deaths worldwide, comparable to the Spanish flu.

There was still no PPE as recommended by the WHO, so I spent a Sunday morning on eBay trying to find protective disposable suits. They were mostly sold out – though you could still order them from China. And the news from Wuhan was that life in the city was starting up again – its train station opened that weekend, against a background of only 47 new cases, all in people flying in from abroad.

As I drove down empty motorways that weekend on the way to my shift, I saw the notice boards saying simply 'STAY HOME, PROTECT THE NHS, SAVE LIVES'.

As the month drew to a close, the thought of what the virus could do if it got into care homes was terrifying. There was a new drill for visiting Covid-suspected patients in those homes, and we GPs were told at first we could either adopt the protocol for every patient we saw within a care home or just for those with cough and cold symptoms, or fever.

First, we were to phone the care home staff from the car

park before entering, to make sure the issue couldn't be dealt with from outside, and warn them we'd be wearing PPE. I was to ask the staff to bring the patient as near to the door as possible, so that I wouldn't have to walk through the home. I was to stay two metres from the patient until the moment of examination. If possible I was to ask the patient to take their own temperature, and measure their own oxygen levels, by handing over the equipment. I was to keep my examination as minimal as possible, then decide on a patient care plan from outside, after cleaning all the equipment and taking off my mask and apron. All wipes and PPE were to be double-bagged and incinerated, and all medications for the patient left at the front door.

One of my first visits was to a man in his eighties with Parkinson's disease; he had fallen out of bed and wasn't using his arm. I stood in my shirt sleeves, mask and apron on the doorstep of his nursing home, shivering and looking for the buzzer, until I realised that the door was open.

All visiting had been suspended, and the atmosphere inside was sombre: there was a crushing atmosphere of sadness among the residents, many of whom had dementia, not able to understand why their families no longer came to visit. How do you explain social distancing to someone who doesn't remember where they are, sometimes even who they are? The staff, though, were magnificent – through their own masks and aprons they were doing their best to keep to usual routines. But the care home sector has spent decades trying to emphasise the 'home' in 'care home': they are not clinical spaces, they have carpets and soft furnishings, bingo nights and group excursions, dancing and card games. The expectation that a care home could limit the spread of a virus in the same way as a hospital could seemed absurd. Making residents feel at home, looking after them, often with inadequate resources, is an enormous accomplishment, and as ever I stood in awe of the work that carers do. And not for the first time, I thought how much the phrase 'intensive care' might reflect more than the specialist, techno-medical specialism of keeping people alive, but also the kind of attitude that works tirelessly to keep them happy, safe and living with dignity. This care home at least seemed to have plentiful supplies of masks and gloves.

So many door handles to negotiate! So many points of contact: my hand on my patient's shoulder as I steadied him, my bag placed by the bedside table, the thermometer at his ear, the oxygen probe on his finger, my hands on his shoulder as I tested his deltoid muscle, my hands on his elbow as I gently rotated the joint. He hadn't broken anything, and it didn't appear as if his fall was precipitated by an infection or a stroke.

'Any Covid cases?' I asked the shift manager as I gathered my things. She shook her head.

'Not so far,' she said, 'but I've heard some haven't been so lucky.' I'd began to hear the rumours, too – of patients being discharged from hospital to care homes, bringing the virus with them.

'Tragic, isn't it,' she said as we walked past the day room towards the exit, all the residents spaced out in chairs two metres apart, the staff moving between them under their layers of clinical plastic.

That day it was announced that a UK doctor had died of the virus – Amged El-Hawrani, an ENT specialist.

PEAK

*'I cannot omit taking notice what a desolate place the
city was at that time. The great street I lived in ...
was more like a green field than a paved street'*
Daniel Defoe
A Journal of the Plague Year

We spend our lives immersed in an ocean of air, barely aware
of the ease with which we draw in portions of sky, hardly
thinking of it as something that we could hunger for. Air, the
most immaterial of materials, our most obstinate tether to
life.

It was April now and, as our experience with Covid-19
accumulated, it was becoming clear that for most people, the
virus barely bothers the lungs: sufferers complain of a dry
cough as the virus irritates the upper airways; lack of smell
as the nose becomes infected; fever as the immune system
confronts the infection. A few people have nausea, vomiting,
even diarrhoea as the virus upsets the digestive tract. Headache is a prominent symptom, and a bone-weary, sagging
exhaustion – sending many to their beds for days.

Some estimates began to put the number who are
entirely asymptomatic, but still able to spread the infection,
at between 30 and 40 per cent. About a week into the illness,
four out of five of those who are symptomatic improve, but
in the remainder something more sinister begins to unfold:

the tissues of the lung thicken as the immune system, in its attempt to flush out the virus, begins itself to irritate and inflame the lung. This process is poorly understood, but its result is well known: what should be the lightest, airiest part of the body becomes sodden with fluid. We often think of lungs as deep inside the body, but in truth the lungs, together with the gut, are where our body meets the outside world – as far as the body is concerned they're external, and their flimsy, folded tissues offer a far greater area of contact with air than our skin. Like the leaves of a tree, our lungs have evolved to mingle and exchange the gases we are immersed in; unlike leaves, they're moist and always warm – an ideal breeding ground for inhaled microorganisms. The immune reaction can make them even more moist, so much so that they can no longer perform their proper task of gas exchange. Covid-19 has been called a 'biphasic' illness because it has two phases: first 'virological', as the virus sickens the body; and then 'immunological', as misdirected messages from the immune system end up hindering rather than helping the lungs.

Heavy, sodden lungs are less efficient, and are difficult to breathe with – people get exhausted, which is why ventilators are needed, to take over the job until the body heals itself. But our lungs didn't evolve to have air blown into them – they evolved to suck air, thanks to the outward motion of the rib cage and the downward motion of the diaphragm as you breathe in. Specialists in intensive care know that ventilators are a poor substitute for natural breathing. Pushing air at force down into the lungs damages them: it stretches some parts as thin as overblown balloons, while other boggy, swollen parts fail to inflate properly. Uninflated parts of lung are like dead weights: they don't help with gas exchange and, just as a stagnant pool is a fertile medium for all kinds of life, stagnant portions of lung are at risk of breeding the kind of bacteria that cause pneumonia. Blowing air into the chest also restricts the heart. The inadvertent damage that mechanical ventilation does to lungs is one reason that I was hearing from colleagues in ITU that 6 out of 10 people with Covid-19 needing ventilation, and a third of those admitted to hospital overall, were dying of the disease. But for the moment, that ventilation was the best option we had, and without it the sickest patients would not have had a chance.

On 1 April, a medical school friend, Colin Speight, sent me a link to a project he was involved in. Colin is a GP now, but in former lives has been a tropical medicine physician, an HIV specialist in Malawi and a keen Antipodean surfer – he's one of life's enthusiasts. Together with a team of engineers and physicians he was involved in developing a new kind of ventilator, one that worked on the same principle as the old 'iron lungs' that helped people survive serious epidemics of polio through the 1950s and 1960s. Polio was known as a 'silent killer'; the causative virus attacked not the lungs but the nerves that made the muscles move. Victims would suffocate not because the lungs thickened and stiffened with the fluid of an immune reaction, but because the diaphragm and chest muscles that sustain breathing were paralysed, albeit temporarily.

An iron lung is in essence a steel cylinder to lie down in, with a tight rubber seal at the neck. It has an outlet for a urinary catheter, and window hatches in the side for toileting. A machine draws air from the cylinder on a timer, creating a vacuum around the body which pulls the chest wall outwards to produce breaths. Air pulled, rather than forced, into the lungs is less damaging; some patients have remained in iron lungs for decades at a time.

The iron lungs being developed now by the 'Exovent' team are shorter, and sit over the trunk only – they have neoprene seals at the neck and around the abdomen. Patients can remain conscious on them, and are able to eat and drink – something that is impossible with traditional tube ventilation, where a wide-bore tube sits in your throat. The clinical staff need less specialist training to manage such patients and, when in motion, the machines create fewer sprayed droplets of virus than other ventilation methods. Breathing through suction rather than blowing helps, rather than hinders, the pumping action of the heart. The project is a not-for-profit humanitarian endeavour, with no financial reward for anyone involved – the team hoped to create a version of the machine for low-to-middle-income countries that would cost only £200 to produce.

Ancient ideas proposed the body as a fusion of water and earth, with air a kind of vital energy needed to ignite the flame of life. In April, as the virus fanned out through the population, hospitals began to fill up with people struggling for breath, their lungs drowning in fluids that threatened to extinguish that flame. It seemed difficult to believe that for all our technomedical sophistication, we were having to repurpose old ways of accomplishing that most primitive and basic of physical functions, the bringing of oxygen to the struggling membranes of the lungs.

On 3 April the UK Prime Minister, Boris Johnson, at home self-isolating with coronavirus, posted a video online. For a doctor it was alarming to watch: he was visibly overbreathing, interrupting his sentences to take brief gasps. Two days later he was admitted to hospital, and on 6 April to Intensive Care. The country itself seemed stunned; no other national leader had yet been affected by the virus so severely. The Foreign Secretary took over press briefings. The BBC published flow charts of how power would transition should the Prime Minister die, which seemed at first premature, but then perhaps there was a need to reassure people that anarchy wouldn't descend on the country. The weekend came: Scotland's Chief Medical Officer, Catherine Calderwood, was spotted visiting her holiday house after fronting the media campaign telling everyone else not to. By Sunday night she had resigned, and her deputy, Gregor Smith, had taken over as interim CMO.

Worse stories emerged from Italy. My wife heard of a social club in Lombardy frequented by the father of a childhood friend: not long before Italian lockdown had been implemented an event had brought seventy people together from all corners of the province. One of them must have had the virus, because of the seventy who gathered that day, forty were now dead.

By the end of the first week of April, into the third week of UK lockdown, we were reaching our first peak of patients requiring ITU. Each day I'd watch the figures on my NHS computer screen, my fingers trembling as they clicked between graphs of thin blue lines in steep ascent. London was emerging as the centre of the UK's epidemic: hospitals were closing there for lack of oxygen, while in Edinburgh each day brought thirty to forty more people into hospital with Covid pneumonia – an admission rate that couldn't be sustained for long. I wondered whether the hospital, too, would have to close, and we'd be forced to shunt patients to the new one, hastily erected in the SEC Centre in Glasgow, now named the NHS Louisa Jordan, for a Scots-Irish nurse celebrated for her work in the First World War. One of the drivers for the evening and weekend service asked me what I thought of the rumours, circulating on the internet, that the virus was manmade. I told him that as conspiracy theories go it was absurd: why would any government make a virus that is utterly uncontrollable, that has no respect for borders, that could so swiftly debilitate an economy? He didn't look convinced; perhaps suspicion is hard-wired into us. In the 1600s an English physician, Thomas Browne, wrote of a manmade plague sweeping through Milan, that 'allegedly was induced by a powder and a pestiferous ointment'.

Reports on the Prime Minister's progress were anodyne and bloodless, as if the hospital spokespeople had something to hide. At the same time, in my day to day work the pandemic felt like a flu outbreak: I was speaking to three or four patients with Covid symptoms each day, but almost all of them were managing at home – even those with underlying health conditions such as asthma and diabetes. I wasn't having to admit any to hospital.

The sickest patients were directed to the Covid Assessment Centre for a face to face assessment. The response to the call for volunteers had been good and, despite my offer of working Thursdays and Sundays, there were only a few shifts on the current rota where I'd be needed.

Training as a GP emphasises the importance of building empathy and rapport, but on shift in the Covid hub I stayed as far from the patients as possible until the moment of actually examining them, even taking their medical history from the far side of the room. I remember seeing an overweight middle-aged man there who had flown in from Italy not long before lockdown. Another who had caught it at his mother's funeral, just as one of my own patients had caught it at a funeral (it seemed the ongoing restriction of numbers at burials and cremations was a cruel necessity). A builder who'd had a sick workmate on the last site he'd worked at before lockdown. A young mother who thought she'd caught it on the train from London. On shift one Thursday evening we all stopped at 8 p.m. to listen for the sound of clapping to celebrate health care workers, but the clinic is surrounded by hospital buildings, and the night was silent. 'It makes my toes curl anyway,' said one of my colleagues. 'I'll be glad when it stops.'

'I like it,' I said. 'It's the one time of the week I get to see all my neighbours.' For me, those Thursday rituals were far more about people cheering one another on than about thanking the NHS.

In my area of Lothian there are usually two cars providing emergency GP home visits over the weekends and in the evenings. A few days after Boris Johnson was admitted to hospital, I was out in 'Car 2', driving to the most urgent triage category of visit – which means getting there within an hour. On the phone, the patient had said that after a week of flu-like symptoms he was breathless even lying on his sofa, and had a fever – a characteristic story, and I knew that thousands of visits like this one were going on every day, up and down the country. It was early evening, westering sunlight was turning the suburban streets golden, blackbirds were singing in privet hedges. I phoned the patient from the car for directions. His breath came in gasps, his sentences interrupted.

'Are you alone?' I asked. 'Yes.' 'Can you sit near the door?' 'Yes.' 'Just to warn you, I'll be wearing an apron, mask, visor, gloves. I'll give you a mask and gloves to wear, too.' 'OK.' 'If you sit near the door, it's easier for me – I won't have to come all through the house to find you.' 'OK.'

I ignored the twitching curtains of the neighbours, the kids out on their bikes. Earlier in the shift, leaving another home visit, a patient had asked me, 'Can you shout to the neighbours that I *don't* have Covid?' Now I stood at the back of the car, opened the boot, and began the Great Faff, another new protocol to get accustomed to. Thermometer, oxygen sensor, stethoscope, all placed into a clean, clear plastic bag.

Apron on, mask on, gloves on, then a second pair of gloves over the first. The apron flapped about in the wind. Some of my colleagues have been Sellotaping the thin flapping plastic to their legs, or using bulldog clips. Visor on last – its frame was 3D-printed in green plastic, with clips for attaching a head strap to the back, and a clear acetate shield to the front. On the inside of the forehead band was written 'Car 2' in Magic Marker.

At the patient's front door, which was ajar, I breathed in the smell of stale cigarette smoke. The man was sitting on a stool just inside the door, elbows on his knees, bracing his chest with his arms to better move air in and out of his lungs. He was wearing grey pyjamas that had lost a couple of buttons.

'How are you doing?' He grunted an acknowledgement. 'Can you manage to put on one of these?' I handed him the mask, but he couldn't tie the strings of it. Wishing my forearms weren't bare, I leaned over him, holding my breath, and knotted the ties at the back of his head and neck.

I counted his breathing – fast, at 28 breaths per minute – and a digital thermometer in his ear flashed red with an impressive fever. I put an oxygen sensor over his finger – by shining light through the skin it gauged the oxygen content of his blood, which was worryingly low. His pulse, as he sat on the stool, was galloping along at more than 2 beats a second.

'Can you stand up for me?' I asked. We shuffled awkwardly in the small hall in a doleful dance; he turned around and I lifted his pyjamas to place my stethoscope on his back. The sound of the air passing through his lungs was accompanied by a quiet hissing sound, like sizzling fat. The sound of pneumonia. In his case, pneumonia probably caused by Covid-19.

'I'm going outside then I'll phone you about what

happens next,' I told him. I picked up the clear bag with my stethoscope, oxygen sensor and thermometer, and stepped out, trying to hold central to my awareness and every action that there was virus on the walls of the house, on the door handle, on my gloves, and on all my equipment.

On the doorstep I gulped down the fresh air, then it was back to the rigmarole: topmost layer of gloves off and into a waste bag. With my underlayer of gloves I took a chloride wipe and began to clean all the equipment – stethoscope, oxygen sensor, thermometer – and placed them into yet another clear plastic bag, ready for the next patient. The wipe went into the waste, then my apron. Next it was the visor's turn to get cleaned, and afterwards I placed it on the ground to dry. Then undergloves off, mask off, the clinical waste bag tied off and sealed, and it was back into the car.

With all this donning and doffing of PPE, and cleaning of all the equipment, home visits now took far longer than they used to. I'd have been much happier wearing a gown in addition to the gloves, mask and visor – it would have better protected my arms, trunk and legs from droplets of virus. But, for now, there were no gowns available. A few days earlier I had looked through the supplies of gloves and masks that had been delivered to my practice from central government stores: the masks were stamped with the name of a Canadian company, manufactured in China, and distributed by yet another company from Germany. My gloves had all been manufactured in Malaysia or Vietnam. If we were to get this equipment to the people who needed it in the UK, we needed manufacturers here – and production should have started in January.

From the car I dialed the man's number again; all those years learning about personal consultation styles, and now I was breaking bad news by telephone from a car parked outside my patient's house. As I waited for him to pick up I glanced at the car mirror; my forehead was stamped with 'Car 2' in reverse, transferred in sweat from the visor headband.

'I think it's likely that you have coronavirus,' I heard myself say, 'and that it's affecting your lungs, causing pneumonia. That's why you feel so breathless.' Silence. 'I'll arrange for an ambulance to come and take you to hospital.'

I waited. His breathing was audible. 'Is there anything you'd like to ask?'

'How long for?' he said.

'I don't know.'

Heading on to the next patient I passed the ambulance I'd just called, on its way to collect him. The paramedics both waved and I waved back – one, who wasn't yet wearing his mask, smiled. One of the few consolations of this pandemic is its grim camaraderie, a new fellowship among the fear.

Later I walked from the GP clinic to the A&E department to see how my patient had fared. One of the emergency nurse practitioners called up his X-ray on the screen: lungs should be light and spongy, the blackness of air clear against the white of ribs, diaphragm and heart. But an 'infiltrate' had clouded his lungs; where there should have been a black void there were speckled galaxies of white.

'How old is he?' the nurse practitioner asked me.

'Mid-fifties' I said. 'Like the Prime Minister.'

'Overweight?' I nodded.

'They're all like that, up in ITU,' she said. 'Strange days.' We paused together for a moment in silence in front of the X-ray, before she had to go and attend to another patient, and so did I.*

*

---

*He survived, and was discharged five weeks later, having spent just under a week in ITU.

It was striking how many more people were out and about during the day than usual, now that so many were 'working' from home, furloughed, or rendered redundant – free to take walks whenever they liked. At the supermarket the evening queue snaked across the car park, everyone two metres apart; on entering we had our hands sprayed with sanitiser before being offered a freshly wiped shopping trolley. Progress through the supermarket was via a one way system, with no one supposed to go near anyone else. We were all potential assassins now.

Some clip-together disposable goggles arrived at my own clinic in an unmarked bag, but they were fiddly to put together and easily fell off – instead, we ordered wipe-down visors from an online DIY store. There had been media reports of staff being reduced to using kids' ski goggles and having to wear bin bags – according to the news, many nursing homes were entirely without PPE. An official diktat arrived that any 'home-made' PPE should not be used unless it has been subject to safety assessments. The authorities, it seemed, didn't want people taking their safety into their own hands, but without adequate provision, what choice did carers have?

New guidance was sent out to every medical practitioner in Lothian urging us *not* to shy away from difficult conversations. For GPs, discussions about 'rationing' healthcare are nothing new, but I had the sense that society was only just becoming aware of the gruelling questions that, within medicine, we're accustomed to asking. Difficult conversations about whether or not to admit frail older people to hospital didn't begin with Covid – for GPs, they're a daily reality.

One of the guidance documents described how under 'surge conditions' it might become necessary to review all patients in the ITU every twenty-four hours and make a clear decision as to whether they were truly benefitting, and reminded me that the over-seventies have a very low success rate from ventilation and that the use of ITU would need to be 'optimised'. In other words, I should prepare myself to tell patients, or their families, that there was little point referring the majority of frail older people to hospital even if they wished to be. Cynics pointed out that this seemed more a question of resources than anything else – not enough staff or ventilators to go around. True, but at the same time, overly simplistic: so few people with Covid-19 were surviving ITU that raising hopes of patients and families, only for them to die in a place where visitors weren't allowed, would also bring cruel and unnecessary suffering. The advice closed with a long and very helpful appendix setting out the kinds of morphine and sedative doses we might need to assist those dying of Covid pneumonia at home.

As hospitals were weighing up the best way to help failing lungs draw breath, GPs like me were contacting everyone on our patient lists who fell into a vulnerable category, asking them to 'shield' themselves from the virus until July at least. It was as dismal a task as it was important, and I made the calls with a heaviness of spirit that I tried to disguise. It felt wrong to have such a distressing conversation on the phone, condemning each new patient to a kind of voluntary imprisonment. The categories included organ transplant recipients, those on active treatment for specific cancers, those with severe lung disease, the significantly immunosuppressed, and pregnant women with underlying heart problems. A further catch-all category was added to include anyone else GPs deemed vulnerable. My colleagues and I spent a fortnight going through lists of patients, doubling the number eligible for 'shielding' and passing their details to the government: everyone in the category was given a code which offers priority for supermarket food deliveries, benefits and community support.

I spent hours on the phone each day. Many of my patients were deeply frightened, and my line of questioning didn't help. Did they understand the official advice? Did they need any assistance? Were they happy for the hospital and paramedic staff to have access to a summary of their medical history? Could we update their next of kin details? Grim stories emerged of GPs cold-calling patients to ask whether they wanted resuscitation attempted should they succumb to coronavirus, but I never broached those discussions unless someone raised it themselves. A study was circulated showing that around one in three people appreciate an invitation to have that kind of impromptu life or death conversation, but for the majority it was either unwelcome, insensitive or irrelevant.

In the case of pneumonia from Covid-19, 'irrelevant' was almost certainly true. Cardiac resuscitation can be helpful to restart a stopped heart after sudden, temporary interruption in its rhythm, but when the heart stops because of Covid-19 pneumonia it's practically useless. Mechanical analogies of the body are rarely accurate – who ever heard of a turbine healing itself? – but in this case those analogies hold true: CPR for Covid-19 pneumonia would be like fixing a starter motor when the engine has already broken down.

The number of sick patients was rising in a straight line, with about 1,000 new cases testing positive every day across the UK, despite the lockdown. A huge number of NHS services were on pause, but of course anything related to births or deaths carried on regardless. We had the same number of phone calls from women who were pregnant as we always did, asking advice and for referral on to midwives. The lockdown had been effective in slowing spread and, at the level of our own practice ,we had about the same number of people dying as usual, and were making just as many palliative care visits to help those at the end of life stay at home if they possibly could.

One patient in particular I remember from that time, a man in his nineties, Mr Donaldson. He had a chronic distrust of doctors, or rather of medications, and we'd joked often over the years about his reluctance to have his aches and pains, his heart trouble and his blood pressure adequately treated. Often on my visits I'd sit on his sofa as he watched the lunchtime news and we'd exchange opinions about politics. On the NHS, he'd say, 'I thought it a good idea – I remember voting for it!' On Brexit, he'd say, 'That Boris Johnson, he's a maverick, an entertainer.' Now he was dying, of some silent cancer that together we'd decided not to identify or pursue, because he didn't want to go to hospital and didn't believe knowing the name of his disease would be any comfort to him. Whatever it was that was killing him would be allowed to continue unimpeded; he'd be spared the indignities of tests and clinic rooms for the sake of dying swiftly and, we hoped, in peace. 'This is no life anyway,' he'd say.

I thought of how few nonagenarians I knew who still enjoyed a good quality of life, and the bleak sadness of being in the last weeks or months of life but told to isolate from their wider family, and from society. It seemed one of the cruellest corollaries of the measures we had taken as a society, and every day brought new conversations with lonely old people who, week after week, saw no one but paid carers. That the virus spreads through speech and through touch was one of its harshest twists, attacking the most basic elements of our humanity – how we connect, empathise and show love.

My visits to Mr Donaldson often coincided with those of one of the district nurses, Michaela, whose efforts kept him as comfortable as was humanly possible: like so many of the other medical professionals I work with, a true provider of intensive, compassionate long-term care. On those shared visits Michaela and I would gently roll him to check his back for sores ('Easy does it there, Mr D!') and try to position him on the hospital bed that had been drafted in to make nursing him easier through those last days. I felt awkward bending over the bed in apron and gloves and peering at him through an acetate visor, but he didn't seem to mind. 'I'm surrounded by kindness,' he muttered, asking us again and again to keep him comfortable and out of hospital. His voice was a whisper, but his last words to me were: 'This bloody virus.'

Before the pandemic, whether in ITU or out in the community, every day in medicine was a mixture of triumph and tragedy. In the thick of that first peak through April my days felt much the same, though conducted through a strange, sad and impersonal barrier of PPE and phone calls, and being able to see so few of my patients face to face. With my colleagues in the practice the jokes, puns and anecdotes continued: there can be great fellow feeling between colleagues in such an intense environment. As we peered at one another from behind masks and visors, we found ways of reminding ourselves what we love about the work, reassuring one another that the pandemic would eventually pass and the community would recover.

The mental health consequences of this crisis were deepening: some days every call I took was about loneliness, self-harm, anxiety, panic attacks. France was arranging hotel rooms for victims of domestic abuse forced into staying home with violent partners. New infections in Italy were slowing after four weeks of lockdown in some places, but they were not seeing any slowdown in deaths – still 800–900 per day. Russia's cases were climbing fast, Spain's were at 1,000 a day. The UN Secretary General called it the worst crisis since the Second World War, without parallel, while more countries were beginning to report anger against China for not managing to contain the virus. In the US, where the President constantly undermined state-level attempts to enforce any lockdown, case levels were surging past those of China.

More details began to emerge about the stealthy way in which the virus took hold in the body: studies were published that showed that SARS-CoV-2 was four times easier to catch than SARS-CoV-1 had been. The lollipops of sugared protein that jut from the new virus's surface – the 'keys' through which the virus enters human cells – were four times 'stickier'. SARS-CoV-1 readily infected the lungs, while evidence was beginning to emerge that the new one preferred to begin with the upper airway – nose, throat and windpipe. That affinity for the nose and windpipe made it more dangerous, because it could spread more easily through sneezes and nasal drips.

More detail began to emerge about the disparity in the virus's effect between the old and the young: immune studies were published showing that the older someone was, the more likely they were to generate a devastating immune response to Covid in the thick of the second, lung-clogging phase of the illness, when the cells that should protect the body from invasion began instead to attack it. The immune system in the elderly is often less efficient at tackling viruses in the first place, and now it looked as if the elderly were doubly disadvantaged: more susceptible to the virus itself, and more likely to be swept away by the storm of the body's late, damaging response to it. But the pattern was mysteriously uneven – some elderly people showed no response at all, as if they carried in their genetic make-up some as-yet unidentified protection. Every copy of the virus would enter the human body the same way: by applying that lollipop 'key' (the 'spike' protein) to one of many potential 'locks' that cover the cell membranes of human tissue. SARS-CoV-2 binds frighteningly well to one called ACE-2,* which ordinarily helps regulate blood flow through the tissues. Men seemed to be more severely affected by Covid-19 than women, perhaps because they have more ACE-2 coating their body cells; children have much less, offering an explanation for why in general they're so mildly affected.

In mid-April it was confirmed that the virus came directly from horseshoe bats, not through an intermediate species such as pangolins, as had previously been thought. Other viral mapping studies indicated that the virus prevalent in New York seemed to have come from Europe, not Asia, and was circulating widely when I was there back in February – at a time when a China travel ban was in place, but not a European one. I couldn't help thinking of all the hands I had shaken at the New York Academy of Sciences, and wondered if I'd put any of my New York friends at risk. The idea of travelling across the Atlantic already seemed like a strange and remote possibility.

We heard of more deaths in the distance, as rumours. As I passed hours of clinic time on the telephone, talking with people at risk and asking them to 'shield' themselves from this virus, I listened to their stories. In one local family, a middle-aged woman was in ITU with it, and both her elderly parents had already succumbed – one had died in hospital,

---

* Angiotensin Converting Enzyme 2

the other at home. The daughter had been unconscious for a week, and didn't yet know that her parents were dead of an illness she had likely transmitted to them both. Another patient told me of her grandfather, who had been in ITU for ten days before it became apparent that he wouldn't be able to come off the ventilator. Eventually he was allowed to come off the machine and die in a side room.

From rumours, to reality. Miss MacInnes was in her early eighties, a retired schoolteacher, still formidable in her tweed skirts and incongruously dainty hats. For ten years I'd enjoyed her visits: her diatribes about the city council, as much as her lyricism in praise of whatever poetry collection she was currently reading. I'd never had to visit her at home, and so it was a surprise to hear from the receptionist that she'd called for a home visit. Her niece had visited as usual with some shopping and found her muddled: unable to find her way to the bathroom; incapable of preparing a meal.

'Has she had a fever?' I asked. 'A cough?' But no. The niece said that she herself had felt tired, queasy and as if she had a headache a week earlier. But the pain and nausea had left her quickly; she was tired, but was otherwise well.

For a few days my colleagues and I returned to Miss MacInnes's house, trying antibiotics for a presumed urine infection, and seeing if we could get urgent help put in place through social services to assist with her meals. But it was clear that she was becoming more and more unsteady, and would need admission to hospital for round the clock nursing care.

On arrival at hospital, three days after my first visit, she swabbed positive for Covid-19. A week later she died.

The last few hours of life are often peaceful ones, but agitation is not unusual in the days leading up to death. As life begins to unmoor from the body it has often seemed to me as if the body, sensing an ending, begins to lash out, to lay hold of new energy and snatch at what remains of life. This disease is no different – in their agitation some sufferers seem to fight and pull at the very oxygen masks that are keeping them alive.

Miss MacInnes's niece told me that her brothers and cousins were now ill with the virus; that her own parents, themselves very elderly, were in isolation against it. Focussed on their own struggle with fever, breathlessness, exhaustion, it was difficult for her brothers and cousins to grieve. Five would be allowed at the funeral, she told me, and no one would be able to hug one another.

Within the orbit of my practice are several sheltered housing complexes, where people, mostly in their eighties and some in their nineties, live reassured by the proximity of a warden, cheered and supported by a community of others. They have coffee mornings, knitting circles, exercise classes – but everything was cancelled now. Each was confined to their own small room, each fearful, and at my visits I found every one of my patients despondent, even despairing. 'When we want to go sit in the garden,' one told me, shaking her head, 'we have to go one at a time.'

Towards the second half of April Mr Denholm, who'd once had a heart attack and who came into the surgery every few weeks for blood tests, didn't show up for his appointment. Pearl, one of our superb receptionists, asked me if I thought we should be worried. 'He's not answering his phone,' she said. 'That's not like him'.

'Have we got a next of kin for him?' I asked. We didn't.

After a day of calling Mr Denholm, and getting no response, we alerted the police, who kicked in his door. He'd been dead a couple of days, they guessed. Between 3 April and 10 April there were 8,500 more deaths in England and

Wales than in the same period the year before; only 6,000 or so of them were presumed due to Covid-19. Those 'excess deaths' were presumably among people for whom the virus had prevented them getting access to healthcare, either through a diminution of services or because they were too frightened of the virus to go to hospital when they should. I kept returning to the thought that Mr Denholm might have had chest pain in the hours before he died, but didn't call an ambulance for fear of catching the virus.

Much media attention has been paid to doctors, nurses and carers dying of this disease: how inadequate their PPE was; how they were being redeployed in unfamiliar environments; how they were selflessly exposing themselves to the virus in the fulfilment of their vocations. But little has been said about other front-facing, public sector workers such as the police, who were as busy during lockdown as ever, both because of the need to administer it, and because those most likely to break the law were the least likely to observe the restrictions. When I worked regularly in A&E it often felt as if clinical staff and police officers were on the same side, the only sober folk in a city of drunken idiocy. As a GP my encounters with the police are less frequent – I call them if someone in the throes of psychosis is a risk to themself or others, or if, as in the case of Mr Denholm, I can't get access to the home of someone I'm worried about. But I've never forgotten the solidarity of those nightshifts in A&E.

In mid-April I was chatting with a police officer about one of my patients, and heard how difficult the challenges thrown up by the pandemic had been for that service: some stations had been earmarked 'red', for potential Covid positive offenders – those with fever or symptoms – while other stations were presumed 'green' or 'clean'. But how this was to be determined, let alone enforced, was an open question: police officers have to arrest people, often wrestle and restrain them, all the while at risk of being coughed at in the face. We'd seen within medicine that those who intubate, examine throats, perform endoscopies were at much higher risk of catching the disease, though I've heard little discussion of the risks of wrestling someone to the ground in order to handcuff them. Hot-desking in the back offices of police stations is common, too – another risk factor for transmission. We were all going to need better masks, millions upon millions of masks.

On 15 April the global number of confirmed cases passed 2 million, and would reach 3 million before the end of the month. Forecasts suggested the global economy had already shrunk by 3 per cent, and carbon emissions were set to fall by 8 per cent – for the first time reaching a level that experts estimated is needed year on year to meet international targets. It was being reported that the Himalayas were visible from Delhi, and in Venice the canals were running beautifully clear. But no one was out enjoying the clearing airs and waters. Friends around the country who lived in tourist hotspots told me how wonderful it was to have the place to themselves, though that sensation was bittersweet: their local economies were crumbling, with no prospect of alternatives to be found.

Edinburgh's Royal College of Physicians was running an online series of seminars, and I logged on to hear a Professor of Emerging Infectious Diseases and Global Health at Oxford, Peter Hornby, updating the College on one of the first research trials to combat Covid-19. It was the RECOVERY

Trial, comparing different medications: hydroxychloroquine; an antibiotic called azithromycin; two anti-virals; and steroids – drugs that reduce the intensity of the body's own immune response. The trial was building on some of the research conducted in China early in the Wuhan outbreak, which suggested antiviral drugs may have some promise. There had been a fanfare of publicity around the use of hydroxychloroquine, but the results so far had been disappointing.

In Lombardy, where the first peak had passed and the grip of the virus on the population was in decline, the provincial government issued my mother- and father-in-law with a surgical mask each, to reduce their risk of inhaling particles of virus. Everyone in Italy was to wear a cloth mask of some kind or another, to minimise spread by those carrying the virus rather than to prevent inhalation of it. By the end of April the same advice was issued in Scotland, and hastily prepared home-made masks began to appear around the city.

One of the acute hospital physicians, Claire Gordon, wrote a document that was circulated to us GPs towards the latter half of April that underlined just how protean and unpredictable the manifestations of the virus could be, which in their diversity, and their severity, seemed so much more extreme than any other viral disease I was accustomed to treating. 'Fevers I have seen with Covid are pretty mind-blowing in terms of height and duration,' Gordon wrote, expressing the surprise many of us had felt assessing these coronavirus patients. 'Paracetamol barely touches them.' The breathlessness was often subtle, and patients were frequently unaware of just how unwell they were until they tried to move, and found themselves gasping for breath. When considering whether people might be ready to go home, she was monitoring patients' oxygen levels while walking to and fro in the ward – those in whom oxygen levels dropped on minimal exercise would have to stay in.

As I'd seen for Miss MacInnes, for many elderly people
the only sign of infection was feeling muddled, taking to
bed, while younger folk complained of muscle pains or a sur-
prisingly deep fatigue. Dr Gordon supposed that the older
patients were 'less surprised to feel like they've been run
over by a bus'. Headaches could be so severe that she'd had
to scan Covid patients' brains to rule out haemorrhage; on
the other hand, she said, a common presentation is solely of
nausea and loss of appetite, while 30 per cent of patients have
loss of smell and taste. Numbness of skin and weakness of
muscles could mimic spinal cord disease, and in a few she'd
seen the heart muscle and coronary arteries affected. 'You
may have already picked up that the swab doesn't seem that
reliable yet,' she concluded. 'We're going with gut instinct/
clinical probability based on a lot of the above.' There were
hints about the virus's effect on the body circulation – some
patients developed enormous clots, or 'thromboses', that
seemed to have come out of nowhere, while some patients
of mine with Covid-19, who didn't need to be admitted to
hospital for a cough or for breathlessness, developed odd
rashes suggesting alteration in blood flow to the skin. I
had the fierce awareness that so many of our guesses and
assumptions about this disease and how to tackle it would
seem laughably inaccurate in the years to come – we were
fighting this virus blindfolded by ignorance.

At the same time, it was obvious that in the wider community lockdown was helping slow transmission enormously.
The numbers in ITU dropped consistently from a peak in
mid-April. We GPs were sent a message of praise from the
hospital, thanking us for doing so well at keeping people
away. But it was becoming more difficult to field patient
frustration at the shutting down of much of what the NHS
used to do: no outpatient clinics, no colonoscopies, no IVF,
no ultrasound scans. Even cancer services had been stripped

back to essentials, and many routine lab tests had been cancelled to create capacity for coronavirus testing.

Though the lockdown had cut transmission it was provoking a silent epidemic of despair: panic and anxiety are the virus's dark refrains, a second pandemic leaching into everyone's lives. As the weeks wore on, I was speaking with ever-increasing numbers of people whose mental health, perhaps already fragile before the pandemic, was in freefall. One woman whose mood swings I had supported over the years through face to face conversations, recommendations of long walks, suggestions of group activities and distraction techniques, was now on the phone to me almost daily as we tried new sedative drugs to quiet her seething mind. Another who had only the most tenuous of holds on reality seemed to have drifted off into a world of his own – without the anchors of family, support workers and occupational therapists, his paranoias were deepening and his hallucinations were becoming more frightening. All this while long-stay mental health hospitals – institutions custom-made for viral spread – were still trying to empty their patients into the community 'for their own safety'.

Alcohol-induced injuries in the over fifties were up, as were injuries from assaults. Within our area of the city we already knew of suicides triggered as a consequence of bankruptcies and business closures, and marriages breaking down. Between 23 March and 12 April there were sixteen deaths from domestic violence in the UK – more than triple the still-shocking average in the same period over the last few years. A police officer friend told me that domestic abuse lines were experiencing a 30–40 per cent increase in traffic. The Samaritans and Childline, too, were receiving high volumes of calls. A domestic abuse hotline for NHS workers had been inaugurated – intended to support both health workers at risk and to offer advice should they suspect patients were being abused. When I checked routine blood tests on my patients I was seeing new flares of liver irritation, suggesting rising alcohol abuse.

For those whose jobs offered identity and a sense of purpose, being furloughed was experienced as a tragedy exacerbated by forced disconnection from friends and family, even if others were starting to look on the lockdown as a time of recalibration, and reorientation of priorities – no alarm clocks, no social demands and, for those with relative financial security, an odd fusion of heightened and diminished stress. Many children, my own included, were desperately missing the structure and social life offered by school, and every day I heard of more best-laid plans being added to the bonfire of this global crisis. Home-schooling was proving almost impossible for us, as for so many others – the two days per week I was home caring for my own kids I'd sit with them in the mornings, reading through grids of tasks sent in by their teachers: researching polar bear biology, or the social geography of Northern Ireland, or songs to remember the eight times table. But by noon all three children would be jumpy and distracted, and I'd have to get them out to defuse the tension and tear around the garden in what seemed perpetually glorious sunshine. The UK was experiencing its sunniest April on record, with more hours of sunshine than are normally seen in June or July. At least we have a garden, I thought – small mercies.

A morning clinic, only one patient came in to see me – the rest were dealt with on the phone. It was a man complaining of weight loss, and already it felt like a luxury to be able to assess a patient face to face. One woman told me on the phone of her two sons, one in London, the other in Milan, and how both lost their sense of smell and taste at the same time. They flew back home to be with her in Edinburgh as soon as they had recovered, and only now, four weeks on, did she feel as if she was catching the virus. She felt breathless even walking across her kitchen.

Another patient that day, aged 90, had lived through the war; she told me this lockdown felt worse – much worse. 'I was young then, I know,' she said, 'and the war was far away. But we could get out, meet friends, go to theatres, the cinema! But this …' Words failed her. 'It's just *so hard* for any of us to make one another feel better.' She told me that every day she climbed up and down the stairs in her home a hundred times, trying to keep fit. 'The War was six years, the Spanish flu was two years,' she said to me. 'How long do you think this will go on for?'

I shrugged. 'A couple of years?'

'And I think we need ration books again – that was a fairer way of doing things.'

In an evening Zoom meeting, with 330 Lothian GPs on a single call, I reflected on the birth of a new kind of art form, the simultaneous transmission of so many people's studies, kitchens and living rooms, so many shelves, maps and art works, so many faces reacting to a speaker's presentation. We theorised that more people could die of non-Covid disease, through being unable to access healthcare, than could conceivably die of Covid pneumonia. 'This is the new normal,' the chair said – the phrase we were hearing so often it had been drained of any power. 'We need to explore ways of doing work remotely from our patients.' One of the salient points of the meeting was that, after some fierce lobbying from the medical unions, death in service benefits had been extended to all GPs, in order to persuade us to work in Covid clinics.

The care homes I'd been visiting had all taken extraordinary steps to protect their residents from the virus – the staff within them had changed the way they work, reorientating their domestic geography to keep residents in their rooms as much as was humane. In the three I visit regularly there had been just a handful of cases, and some deaths among residents that had been particularly frail or vulnerable. But we'd been in lockdown now for a month and many GPs were beginning to draw breath, take stock and reach out to one another, and I heard about others who were not so fortunate. In the evening and weekend service, I'd been encouraged to swab any care home residents who seemed symptomatic. Many of my colleagues expressed their unease at being asked to perform such an invasive test, with frightening implications for any home in which a positive case was found, without the PPE recommended by the WHO. On weekend duty I visited homes where exhausted nurse managers spoke of how bewildering their jobs had become – of homes where a worker had swabbed positive, but every resident stayed negative, and others where several residents caught the virus but all stayed well. I listened with horror as a colleague told me of a home neighbouring her own practice where every resident had become infected. In the space of a few short weeks, a third of them had died.

This was the week the US President suggested putting bleach and disinfectant into the blood to combat coronavirus, and trying to get sunlight 'inside'. It was reported on 25 April that thirty people in New York had been hospitalised after following his advice. 'Trump's briefings are actively endangering the public's health,' said Robert Reich, a professor of public policy at the University of California, Berkeley. 'Listen to the experts. And please don't drink disinfectant.'

By 26 April Wuhan had reported that there were no Covid-19 patients left in any of its hospitals – and China as a whole reported its eleventh consecutive day with no coronavirus deaths. Spain's deaths dropped to 288 per day, the lowest since 20 March, while globally the death toll passed 200,000. UK deaths had passed 20,000, but it was broadly recognised that this was an underestimate, given that so many in community care homes hadn't been counted. And in the last days of April the First Minister of Scotland, Nicola Sturgeon, announced a 'decision framework' for finding our way out of lockdown, just as Boris Johnson recovered sufficiently to move back into Downing Street and attend the birth of his son; something many parents in other areas of the country had not been allowed to do.

At this point, the end of April, the R_0 or 'reproduction number', of the virus – how many people each infected person would pass the disease on to – was between 0.6 and 1.0: at this level, cases would continue to drop. But it would only remain so low because of the restrictions; as soon as they eased it was clear that the figure would begin to rise again.

Ramadan began. I took a walk at lunchtime from my clinic to the nearest post box, taking the practice official mail, as well as cards from my kids to their grandparents – they'd leave them untouched for three days after receiving them, to make sure there could be no active virus on their surfaces. And I could feel a change in the air, an impatience – the streets were getting busier, and people more restless.

PART II

REFLECTION

DECLINE PHASE

'[H]e began now to hope, nay, more than hope,
that the infection had passed its crisis and was
going off; and accordingly so it was …'
Daniel Defoe
A Journal of the Plague Year

It's a twelve-mile bike ride from my home to the clinic; I leave the house at around 7.30 a.m. and pedal along a path that in wartime was a railway, but is now a tarmac avenue of holly and hawthorn, alder and elder. On a stretch of the path that runs along the canal I'd seen swans nesting through April; now in May they had six cygnets, and each morning I'd watch them scrambling for their parents' backs at my approach. At the outset of lockdown the path was busier than usual, as people unaccustomed to being home on week-days took the chance to make use of it. By May the novelty had worn off, and I again had the path to myself.

During the first week of May I stopped at a traffic light not far from the surgery. There was no traffic, and it seemed odd to have to wait. A few feet to my left, approaching the crossing point, a woman in a pink mac and checked skirt stumbled on a paving stone and fell to the ground. I began to heave my bike off the road towards her, but a young couple in running gear doubled back and put out their hands to help her before I could get there. She flushed red and repeated,

'I'm fine, I'm fine', seeming both embarrassed and shocked by the offer of personal contact. She hesitated to be helped – public touch being already so rare, almost unimaginable, but then with reluctance stretched out her hand.

A few hundred yards on, at yet another traffic light, I found a startled-looking man laying on his back in his Lycra, his bike on top of him. He'd clipped a roadwork sign with his handlebars and fallen: he, too, was apologetic, and insisted to me that he didn't need any assistance to get back on his feet – he didn't want me to reach out my hand to touch him. 'I'm fine, I'm fine,' he said, though he didn't look it.

How many of us are stumbling and falling these days, I thought, and how many are unable to ask for help?

A few days into April, Mr Mirandola, the elderly Italian gentleman who had told me back in March that the virus was Mother Nature's way of clearing out the oldies, had a heart attack. He was almost cleared out himself: the day he had the heart attack he struggled to use the phone, and fell. Fortunately, he was wearing an alarm button and managed to raise a community alert worker, who called us and we arranged an ambulance.

The day he was released from hospital he called me: 'When are you coming to see me?' he asked. His voice was slightly slurred, and I wondered if he'd also had a small stroke. 'I'm supposed to keep any visits to a real minimum now, Mr Mirandola,' I said. 'So that you're protected, in case I'm carrying the virus.' 'I understand,' he said. 'But when are you coming to see me?'

'Soon,' I replied; I needed to check how his blood pressure, liver and kidneys were bearing up under all the new tablets he'd been put on, in the hope of preventing further heart attacks. He'd always been circumspect about taking any medicines – over the years I'd tried to persuade him of the merits of several, but so far I'd always respected his choice not to take them. This is the kind of care general practitioners can excel in – building a relationship over years, knowing our patients well enough that personal choice, as much as checklist protocols, can guide the treatment.

Mr Mirandola had been a youth during the Second World War, and Jewish – he remembers having to hide from the fascists, how he and his family would live rough in the hills for months at a time. 'I didn't eat bread for months,' he told me. 'I didn't have any shoes.' The triumph of the Allies in the war kindled in him an affection for Britain – he'd lived and worked in Scotland for sixty years now, all within the same kilometre of land. 'Scotland has been good to me,' he said.

On his doorstep I put on my apron, mask, gloves and visor. Many of his carpets had clear plastic protectors over them, dimpled and ridged, and they crinkled as I walked. The flat was pristine – precisely the kind of place the exacting hotelier Mr Mirandola had once been would keep for himself, with dried flowers in vases, some framed prints, professional photographs of his grandchildren. On the coffee table was a printout from the physiotherapists, with stick diagrams showing how he was to exercise his hips, thighs, shoulders, chase the stiffness of hospital immobility from his limbs. Over the fireplace was a gilt-framed print of one of Canaletto's paintings of Venice.

He sat back, switched off the TV and lifted his hand with the remote to point out of the window at the busy thoroughfare of his city centre street. His children and grandchildren were Scots, with no other home than this city, and he spoke with admiration of the neighbours who helped him, the social work support he'd had, the alarm button that had saved his life after his heart attack. 'How much we owe each other,' I thought, as I listened to him talk. Just as in the Highlands and Islands, their very remoteness had both protected the inhabitants and made them vulnerable, in the cities close community had proven vital in surviving the impact of the virus, just as it seemed to accelerate its spread.

The city of Edinburgh was a pioneer in the kind of public health and community medicine now seen as so vital in the control of this virus, but not until the later eighteenth century. It's a beautiful city: seven volcanic hills stand over a metallic firth, a medieval castle on its central stud of basalt. Scandinavian winds blow in from the east, Atlantic rains sweep in from the west. It's home to between 400,000 and 500,000 people now.*

In its earliest years it must have been a spacious place to live – in the 1100s there were only a couple of thousand people living along the spine of what became its 'Royal Mile', the ridge that extends from the tip of the castle to the palace at Holyrood. Orchards and fields lay to either side of the principal road. Water was carried from springs on the flanks of those hills, and sewers ran into a loch to its north. But where there are people there are rats, and in those days where there were rats there was plague. *Yersinia pestis* is a bacterium carried in the mouth parts of rat fleas. When the rats die the fleas turn to humans, with shattering results.

There were frequent plagues in Edinburgh – the Great Plague of Europe, which is said to have arrived with the Mongol armies via ports of the Black Sea, reached the city in 1349. The sick were boarded out into sheds on the moor near the palace of Holyrood, and shipped off to the quarantine

---

* For a history of public health in Edinburgh, see *Bodysnatchers to Lifesavers: Three Centuries of Medicine in Edinburgh* by Tara Womersley and Dorothy H. Crawford (Edinburgh: Luath Press, 2010).

station of Inchkeith Island, part-way across the firth between Lothian and Fife. There were no 'hospitals' as we understand the word, just monastic houses where the monks would palliate the sick while praying for their souls.

The last great plague of Edinburgh was in 1645 when, it was said, 'scarce sixty men were left capable of assisting in its defence'. Everyone who could leave did so, no doubt carrying their pestilence with them. There was still next to no understanding of contagion and, beyond the rudiments of quarantine, little attempt to prevent the spread of disease.

Edinburgh was then falling behind comparable European cities in the control of infections. Through the 1600s there were regular outbreaks of war across Europe, and able students were often obliged to travel to the Netherlands to study medicine at university – a dangerous and expensive journey. The clique of men then charged with the wellbeing of the city –Edinburgh Town Council – realised that, for the health of its citizens, medicine would have to be taught closer to home.

However, it took until 1726 for the university to open a medical faculty, and three years later the council opened the city's first Royal Infirmary. It had just a few bedrooms (with adjoining marble Turkish baths), and was located south of the Royal Mile, at the top of a rise surrounded by orchards and a botanical garden, where a Blackfriars monastery once stood. The modern city commemorates it with 'Infirmary Street'; a Blackwells bookshop stands there now. The councillors in these years were described by writer and jurist Henry Cockburn as 'omnipotent, corrupt, impenetrable … Silent, powerful, submissive, mysterious, and irresponsible, they might have been sitting in Venice'. But by the 1760s they had transformed health in the city: They had built a second infirmary with over 200 beds, and begun the construction of a New Town with broad Georgian streets and revolutionary, life-extending plumbing and sanitation. The city slowly began to rid itself of what the poet and surgeon Tobias Smollett called its 'stercoraceous odours'.

But much of the city remained a lattice of open sewers ('foul burns'); by 1830 cholera epidemics had reached Edinburgh, transported by the networks of the British Empire. Human, horse, donkey, canine, feline, bovine and porcine faeces were all shovelled towards these burns, which regularly burst their banks. As the nineteenth century wore on, the correlation between poverty and early death – which still holds today – grew stronger.

By 6 May the UK had registered 29,000 deaths from Covid, the highest in Europe. On 7 May the First Minister of Scotland, Nicola Sturgeon, extended lockdown further, shortly after insisting on people wearing face coverings in shared transport, shops and places where physical distancing wasn't possible.

The same day, 10 May, UK Prime Minister Boris Johnson relaxed some lockdown measures for England, encouraging a return to work, but still asking people to avoid public transport; he said that driving to work and to places for exercise would be permitted. The message was no longer 'stay at home' but 'stay alert'. How anyone could stay alert against a virus 0.000012 cm in diameter wasn't clear. I asked a friend who works as an ITU specialist in the English Midlands what he thought of the speech. 'No mention of facemasks in public? Everybody in their cars? I think it's an experiment at the expense of the English.' Nicola Sturgeon made it clear she was unimpressed by Boris Johnson's approach: 'I have asked the UK government not to deploy their "stay alert" advertising campaign in Scotland.' The message in Scotland was not 'stay at home if you can' but 'stay at home full stop'.

But the longing to open society, at least a little, was

irrepressible: in my daily GP work it was ever more obvious that the measures were having devastating social and economic consequences, and I hoped that all the sacrifices my patients were making would be worth it, and this lockdown would be the last. Redundancies, suicides, insomnia and bankruptcies, not to mention the effect on children of having no school structure, no exercise, no communal opportunities to play. Although evictions were currently suspended, unless robust housing legislation was urgently put in place, they would inevitably rise as unemployment soared.

'The best protection against coronavirus is your own front door' was a formula often repeated by politicians during this first lockdown. Each time I heard it there was a silent rejoinder in my mind: what if you don't *have* a front door? The emphasis on 'stay at home' was everywhere – government broadcasts repeated it on TV, on the radio, on info boards over motorways and on social media. To give homeless people a 'home' to shelter from the virus, and to recuperate from it safely, was not only a humanitarian ideal but a public health necessity.

On 23 March the Scottish government, public health officials, charities and local councils had all come together to mitigate the worst of the pandemic's effects on the homeless. The initiative was brokered by the charities Streetwork, the Cyrenians and the Bethany Trust. An eighty-bed hotel ordinarily occupied by well-off tourists was hired by the government and within twenty-four hours, the evening of 24 March, it was full of homeless people, as was a smaller hotel, exclusively for female residents. The winter shelter, which would ordinarily stay open until Easter, had already closed to minimise the spread of Covid-19; a third hotel was opened as a temporary 'night shelter' shortly afterwards. Mobile outreach clinics were set up in each hotel and rapid detox and methadone programmes initiated for those who needed them.

*

On 7 May, I had been due at clinic in the Bethany Trust's hotel, but just before attending I came down with a viral headache and felt weak, nauseated and feverish. Instead of going to the clinic I was referred to the public health department, who phoned me with an appointment for a drive-through test. 'Write your name and date of birth on a piece of paper,' the telephonist told me, 'and also write "I AM GOING FOR A COVID TEST".'

'What do I do with the paper?' I asked.

'If the police stop you, don't open your window, just hold it up,' she said.

The test centre was a deserted college car park. The scene was surreal as I drove along empty streets, with leaden limbs, coasting waves of nausea and nursing a headache that felt as if a tiny maniac was rubbing broken glass along the inside of my forehead. I met a gatekeeper in a hi viz vest and, feeling like a royal petitioner, brandished my piece of paper. She waved me on through a slalom of traffic cones that led me to a Portakabin. I'd seen pictures from South Korea of test takers in Perspex cubicles, their arms jutting from perforations into long rubber gauntlets. But my test taker was in a visor and an ordinary surgical mask; she stood by my car in the same flimsy disposable apron I have for my own work, under which she was wearing a sports jacket. I wanted to ask her about just how exposed she felt, but was silenced by the burden of precautions – my car window closed for our brief conversation, she in her visor and mask. She checked my name and date of birth, then asked me to roll down the window; with a knitting needle of a swab she prodded the back of my throat, until I could no longer resist a gagging cough, then, with the same swab, plumbed the back of my nose. And that was that: window up, slalom of cones, hi viz gatekeeper, and I was back on the road for home.

But not ready for work. Clinicians of all persuasions know the temptation is strong to turn up to work no matter how ill you feel, but a death-reaping pandemic had changed everything, and no one wanted to seed an outbreak. I lay in bed, my bones feeling as if their marrow had been replaced with stone, holding still against each wave of nausea. Colleagues seeing my patients for me sent gently enquiring messages, asking when I thought I might be fit to come back. After forty-eight hours of bed rest a text message arrived: negative. Far slower than the six hours my friend Polly had had to wait in Shanghai, but at least it came.

If doctors or nurses received a negative result, and felt well enough, we were told we could go straight back to work. But there are doubts about the effectiveness of the test –high-quality studies estimate that it's accurate only about 70 per cent of the time. With little choice but to accept the results, we were just hoping that if there's insufficient virus in our throats and noses to detect, then there's insufficient to pass on to others.

A few days later I was back in my own practice. Though I could refer people with suspected coronavirus infection to a Covid hub, that was only possible where the patients could make their own way to the centre. Anyone housebound who was suspected of coronavirus was to be assessed in the usual way, by their usual GP.

Mr Magowan was being treated for a cancer diagnosed not long before Christmas, that much I remembered. I looked up his notes: active chemotherapy had been stopped just as lockdown came in, because his blood counts had dropped so far he'd become defenceless against infection, as well as anaemic. His body, it seemed, had reached the limit of what it could take. The request that I visit him at home came from the receptionists, who had taken the call from his wife. Breathless. Fever. Nausea. Because of the counts and the cancer and the chemotherapy, for the last five weeks he'd been shielding from the virus and his wife had been shielding with him.

I called the couple from the street outside their house, in part to prepare them for my mask, apron and visor, and to advise them that I might have to put a mask on Mr Magowan, too. But I couldn't get past the telecom software they'd had installed against cold callers and marketing companies: 'This number is being screened by Call Guardian,' pronounced a voice from the Home Counties – an unlikely protector of this pebbledash semi in a Scottish housing scheme. 'Please say your name after the beep, followed by hash.'

'DR FRANCIS,' I enunciated in as polished an accent as I could muster, and made an exaggerated and unsuccessful press on the hash button. For the second time, nothing happened.

By the doorstep I dropped my medical case, the sterile wipes for later use on my gear, and the waste bag I'd need for the apron, gloves and mask. I had more luck with the door knocker than I'd had with the phone: Mrs Magowan was opening the door even as I stepped back on to the path, to give her space. A colleague knew the couple better than I did, but I had seen her a little over the years: a dainty, elfin woman with wringing hands and harried eyes, wearing the kind of blue chequered tabard once popular to protect clothes from dust and detergent. Under it she wore an old purple cardigan; like her husband, she was in her early sixties.

'I tried to ring,' I said, 'to warn you about all this gear I've got on.' I briefly indicated my apron and held out my bare arms, the pale bands where my wedding ring and watch had been removed, so as to leave nowhere for the virus to hide. Another reason to speak on the phone was to ask her husband to get as close to the front door as possible so that I could minimise my time and passage through the house. But it was too late for that now.

'We're having terrible bother with the phones,' she said, and wrung her hands again.

'How has he been?'

'Oh terrible, doctor, for a couple of days. Can't eat anything – can't keep it down – and he can't get a breath.'

Before coming out I'd spoken with their daughter, Lorna. For the five weeks of her parents' shielding she'd been leaving shopping bags of food on the front step, ringing the bell with a gloved hand, then jumping back. 'I haven't given him it, have I?' she asked me. 'I've been leaving pictures from my kids in the bags with the shopping. They couldn't have passed it on, could they?'

'No, I'm sure you've been very careful,' I said.

Mother and daughter would shout conversations from the gate to the door, devoid of intimacy, everything overheard by the neighbours. 'You OK?' 'OK.' 'Thanks, love.' 'No problem.' Now, from the entrance hallway, I saw the children's pictures fixed to the nearby kitchen wall: crayoned pastoral scenes with lemon yellow suns, pages cross-hatched with 'X's and 'Love you Grandpa'.

'Lovely pictures,' I said, and for a moment the tension in her face eased.

I went upstairs. There were three doors off the small landing, and from the bottom of the stairs Mrs Magowan shouted to me to go through the one directly in front of me. I knocked my blue-gloved knuckles twice on the door's veneer and pushed it open. Mr Magowan was sitting up in bed, three or four pillows piled against a velour headboard. He had a thin white beard and was wearing a threadbare towelled bathrobe, once white. Above his head were more cards and drawings from his grandchildren.

'Hello, Mr Magowan, sorry about all this' – again I

indicated the kit that protected me, even as it removed any subtlety from our conversation. 'Can I get one of these on you, too?' He was breathing hard and, as I placed the mask over the bridge of his nose and folded the metal strip in it into shape, the papery cloth fluttered up and down with each gasp. 'And can you put these on, too?' I handed him a pair of blue latex gloves. There was a melancholy weariness to his movements as he struggled with the gloves – I imagined his exhaustion at having endured the surgery in February for his cancer, then six weeks of chemotherapy, before all these weeks of lockdown, without seeing his grandchildren, only to come down with a fever anyway. He looked grey with fatigue, with resignation.

His temperature was 39°C – too high – and the oxygen sensor on his finger read six or seven points lower than it should have. But it was his breathlessness that worried me: he was gasping for air as if he were climbing a mountain, when all he was doing was lying in bed. I asked him to lean forward, loosened the bathrobe at his neck and inveigled my stethoscope down his back. There was the now-familiar whispering sound to his lungs with each breath, like an ebbing wave as it dissolves into sand.

New research was appearing that suggested in an unventilated room, where someone has been coughing out the virus, it could hang suspended in droplets for hours, in a deadly, invisible mist. Whether you contract it or not depends on how many active viral particles you inhale – for most viruses that figure is thought to be in the high thousands, but for coronavirus it's thought to be in the hundreds. That was why it was obligatory to keep contact time to a minimum. Yet with the Magowans' phone broken, I had no choice but to begin a conversation about Mr Magowan's wishes there in the room with him, trying to keep my breaths shallow, my mask fitting as tightly as I could get it to my face.

I began slowly, trying to gauge his views on hospitals, on oxygen masks, on chest X-rays and blood tests, on the bewildering, tottering edifice of twenty-first-century medicine that stood ahead of him should we decide to send him in. He'd been through enough chemo to know how it would be: the sleepless nights; the overworked, understaffed nurses too busy to answer his buzzer; the ban on visitors; how the hospital and its rhythms would bear down and begin its gruelling, healing work on him. But he also knew how sweet the flow of oxygen would feel as it poured into his starved lungs; he knew how much better he'd feel to have someone, anyone, help him to the toilet other than his frantic wife. The alternative would be to stay at home, to 'take his chances', and for me to give some antibiotics, some morphine, and come back tomorrow. He was not far into his sixties but, given the severity of his breathlessness, I didn't imagine he'd survive more than a few days. I stepped back, trying to give both of us some distance, and, glancing back, saw his wife standing halfway up the stairs, still kneading her hands.

'I won't be able to go, will I?' said Mrs Magowan. I shook my head.

'I'll go in,' said Mr Magowan, shaking his own head. He looked up from the bedcovers, and there was a steeliness in his expression that I hadn't anticipated. 'I'll take any chance of getting better.'

'The ambulance shouldn't be long,' I said. 'Sorry I've got to be so brief.'

'Of course, off you go.'

And wishing I could have spent longer talking things through with him, I backed out of the room.

Rain was falling. Halfway down the garden path I turned back to speak with Mrs Magowan. I hadn't yet had the chance to take off all the gear, clean it and put it back in my bag. 'I will see him again, Dr Francis, won't I?' she asked.

'I'm sure you will, Mrs Magowan,' I said. I removed the top layer of my gloves, dropped them into the waste bag, took a sterile wipe and began cleaning my stethoscope as I spoke. 'Make sure the nurses have your mobile number, not that faulty phone line. They'll be in touch as soon as they can.'

One day, after finishing my own morning clinic on the south side of the city, I went down to one of the hotels on the north side to meet Streetwork's service manager, Rankin Barr.

Behind the reception desk where hotel visitors once gathered for coffee there were files laid out, boxes of food donations, clipboards, lists of names and tasks being ticked off by a team of five workers, each of whom raised a hand to greet me. Barr, who had a clippered haircut and was wearing a Biffy Clyro T-shirt, jeans and Adidas trainers, gave me a casual, welcoming smile. We bumped elbows rather than shaking hands, and I made a joke about my face mask – some of the residents in the foyer were wearing them, too, though none of the staff were. 'I'll give you a tour,' Barr said.

'Here, this is the assessment room.' Just off the foyer was a bland hotel room upholstered in burgundy. A hair dryer was incongruously wired to the clinic desk, and where the bed should have been there was an examination couch – the glued-on headboard hovering halfway up the wall. 'The GPs do their clinics in here,' Barr said. 'Through the back there's another room where we do the Covid assessments.' He led me across the corridor: the room had been a store at some point, and stacked boxes along one wall were covered with washable decorators' sheets.

'Is this where you do the Covid swabs, too?' I asked.

'No, they're done outside,' Barr said, 'in the wind! Safer that way.'

As we walked along the hotel's corridors, I heard wonder in Barr's voice at how much had been achieved in just seven weeks. One resident had slept in a tent for the best part of a decade, he said. 'He was really claustrophobic – I doubted he'd come in at all. But we persuaded him.' Because of his intense anxiety, the man had been allocated the biggest room in the hotel. 'We had to show him how to use the shower, how to operate the TV. He'd been out so long he didn't even know how to switch on a telly.' Barr shook his head. 'He had tears in his eyes.' He told me of another man who normally sleeps curled up in a wheelie bin, which doubles as transport for all his possessions. 'He's under a roof now for the first time in years.' Of a third who still wouldn't come in because a cat had told him it wasn't safe. 'The workers still go out and check on that guy every night, and are working on him – I still hope he'll come.'

'How many are still sleeping out?' I asked.

'Only between five and ten now across the city, I'd say, People who are either too chaotic for us to handle in a setting like this, or who just refuse, who are too used to life on the street.' Barr told me stories, too, of some of the charity's less successful encounters: three men who'd been ejected for dealing drugs, and others who'd been violent; one who'd needed hospital admission after screaming the place down all night.

'Prisoners are putting our assessment hub as their "address" just to get released,' Barr told me. 'And the prison officers don't check – for them it's just a box to tick. We've even had police and probation officers turning up thinking it's a residence, only to find there's no accommodation there, just an office.'

For the first three weeks Barr didn't leave the hotel. 'At first we knew nothing about them, we had only a name and a date of birth. It was hectic –we had some coming off heroin, we had overdoses ...' His voice trailed off. With the streets empty of pedestrians, begging revenue had collapsed – many of Barr's clients were entering the hotel in a state of acute drug withdrawal, unable to afford their usual fixes. 'There were staff who were clocking off at midnight, unable to get home as there's no public transport, so they too stayed in the hotel.' The night staff was now down to just four – a security guard, two Streetwork workers and a member of the hotel staff – but in the early, turbulent days of the project in March and April, having extra staff around had been vital for keeping the peace.

In the first days of the project there had been pushback from neighbours, understandably unhappy about the change to their street. Barr gave them all his mobile phone number, and asked anyone with concerns to phone him, night or day. We stood on the pavement as we talked; as he brought out a ring of keys, one of the residents came past us, picking up litter as he went. 'He does that several times a day – his way of saying thanks,' Barr said. 'The street is cleaner than it's ever been.'

I wondered how they allocate the different flats and homes they have available. 'At the hub near the Salvation Army hostel we have to do a full assessment of each person's needs, and figure out if there are any behavioural issues. Some have complex needs, and some can be dangerous.'

'Dangerous?'

'Well, mental health issues are severe right now, really severe, I think because of the lockdown. Some people aren't good at taking their medication, and we have some smaller units available for people who wouldn't manage in a setting like this.' He stopped a moment and with a wave indicated the whole sweep of the hotel. 'But we're getting to know them now, after seeing them in their rooms three times a day for seven weeks. Are they able to keep their room clean? Are they able to look after themselves? Have they been in any trouble? Any overdoses, or seizures from alcohol withdrawal? So we gather a thorough history on them, and can allocate far more appropriate accommodation than if we were assessing them cold.'

Listening to the story of Barr's weeks in the hotel it was clear that GPs, district nurses and carers didn't have a monopoly on intensive care in the community – that the work he and his colleagues were putting in had been transformative in the good it had done, and was continuing to do. But at the same time I wondered how sustainable the model was – if after only two days the hotels had filled up. But of the eighty people taken in over those first two days, Barr told me, forty-five had already been moved on to more permanent accommodation, and new homeless residents had come in to fill the vacated places. 'Lots of those presenting now are not your traditional rough sleepers. They're coming from broken relationships, and with lockdown they can't go to family, they can't go to B&Bs.'

Around half the rough sleepers in the city are originally from other EU countries, and at imminent risk of losing their right to be in the UK due to Brexit. 'Half of all our residents are classified as "no recourse to public funds" – they can't get benefits and aren't eligible for housing. They're not registered as UK citizens.' The Streetwork team had been working with an immigration expert to clarify each resident's legal status, and help those stranded without papers and who wanted to go home to do so. Fourteen of the eighty current residents were waiting for a decision by the Home Office. We talked about some economists' dark predictions for the autumn, of the economy going into free fall and of the wave of destitution that would result. Barr had access to a discretionary government fund for 'innovative and creative' solutions to rough sleeping, part of which could be used to repatriate people who needed to get home. 'I've got nine people from

Romania who are just waiting for the airlines to open again,' he said.*

Meanwhile, a vaccination programme had just commenced at the hotel. I said I had heard how difficult it was to implement effective immunisation in such a fluid population. Barr nodded. 'Public health have been trying for years.' It was amazing to see how quickly the challenges of caring for rough sleepers had been overcome in the city, when the political will and funding was there. Impressive, but at the same time sad, given how simple the solution turned out to be. Covid was transforming, reorientating society in ways both good and bad, as if all the old hierarchies were being pushed aside and new possibilities were emerging.

I asked Barr how long he thought he could keep going. 'We've funding for six weeks more at least, and I've had assurances that they'll give me at least a month's notice – a month to find other solutions if the money is going to dry up.' But he was optimistic about the future. 'I sit on a committee of all the housing and homeless charities in Scotland, and Kevin Stewart [Scotland's Minister for Local Government, Housing and Planning] sits in on it. All the years I've been working in housing, we've never had that before, a cabinet minister sitting in on our meetings.'

We were back at the main door. I had a clinic to get back to, and Barr had work to do. 'It's the wee things that have made these weeks so extraordinary,' he said. 'The other day we had a birthday party for someone who has been on the streets since the age of nine. Nine! Rough sleeping or in squats since she was a wee girl.' His face shone. 'You should have seen her face. She'd never had a birthday party before.'

---

* By late August Barr had arranged the repatriation of thirty-six of the hotel's residents.

*

In *A Fortunate Man*, John Berger's account of the life and work of a rural GP, published in 1967, Berger notes how many of the doctor's conversations with his patients begin with 'Do you remember when … ?' Berger said of the GP that 'he represents them, becomes their objective (as opposed to subjective) memory'.

With my patients mostly in hiding from the virus, behind closed doors, understanding their worries and easing their concerns was made so much easier by having worked with the same patient group for over a decade; it was common to hear a phrase such as 'It was five or six years ago, Dr Francis – it's the same thing happening again.' That 'thing' could be a nagging pain in the gut, a rash that plagued the legs, the sly unfolding of anxiety. 'Yes, I remember,' I'd say, and go through the notes to find my own entry. 'I see it – it was 2012, actually.' 'Really? I wouldn't have credited it was that long ago.' And I'd begin to read aloud from my notes. Sometimes the words seemed those of a stranger, and sometimes they'd summon an exact memory of that long-gone exchange: how the light was, what the weather was like outside, the way the patient held themselves on the chair, whether they caught or evaded eye contact. It was a comfort for some patients, I know, to find their memory of that exchange validated by what Berger called 'their objective (as opposed to subjective) memory'. It was a comfort, too, for us both to exchange words from another time, when it was straightforward for them to see me, and we spoke face to face rather than visor to visor or through smartphones.

Berger turned his skills as a critic of art on to the patients he saw over six weeks attending GP clinics, out on home visits, in the surgery waiting room, and what impressed him most was the everyday bravery, and tenacity, that those patients manifested. 'Mostly they proceed with the business of living undaunted,' he wrote. 'The notion of endurance is fundamentally far more important than happiness.'

Sometimes it seems as if general practice offers a series of windows into other people's lives, and that through those windows I can glimpse myriad ways of living, modes of coping, of resilience, that continue in their own way, regardless of global events. Robbie was twelve, he told me, when his dad kicked him out. 'He couldn't handle me,' he said. 'He told me he'd had enough, and I could go and live with my mum.' He'd had nothing to do with his mum until then, and the reunion didn't go well. 'I lasted three or four years with her,' Robbie said, 'but eventually she kicked me out, too.' He went to live in Dundee with a half-sister who was a few years older, and had her own flat; Robbie remembers those years as fairly happy. 'I'd never had a place to rely on before,' he said. 'That was the first.'

He got into selling drugs. At sixteen he and his half-sister were drinking vodka laced with street valium; Robbie passed out on the street, a bystander called an ambulance and he woke up in the hospital. His sister, though, made it home, and that was her undoing – when Robbie reached the flat a day or so later, she was dead in bed.

I looked through his notes. He was born in 2002, when I was working in the A&E department of the local children's hospital. He'd been seen there a couple times as a baby during my time there, maybe even by me – once with a fever and once with a fall – and I thought for a moment of our lives' different trajectories across those eighteen years. But here we were once again, sitting together in a brightly lit, clinical space a few hundred yards from that hospital, and in similar roles: he the patient, now an adult, but still struggling to articulate his distress; me the doctor trying to figure out some acceptable way to ease it.

He'd not long been released back into homelessness from psychiatric hospital, and had a string of court dates in the coming months to keep track of – all delayed by the pandemic. There was a room in a B&B for him to go back to and yes, he reassured me, the door could be locked. At least he wasn't rough sleeping. But the auditory hallucinations that had begun to plague him in adolescence had become louder and more insistent. They sounded like mutterings whispered just out of earshot. 'Evil sounds,' he said, and at times he thought he could make out accusations in them, and insults. 'But they're not real,' he added, eyes wide, voice tremulous. I admired the courage of his firmness on that, and his courage in having sought help. Professionals and institutions clearly hadn't helped him much in the past.

'What are you taking?' I asked. Crack, MDMA, Valium, heroin, all in the past week, and he had taken a dose of amphetamine just to get himself to this appointment. 'I think about killing myself every day,' he said, and had scars at his jugular to prove it. He'd been experimenting with overdoses but he must have known, by now, how much it takes to kill and, despite his guilt over his sister's death, the violence of his self-damage, the fact that he'd learnt so young how unreliable people can be, that chaos and uncertainty can break in and destroy anything patiently built, there was something in him that wanted to live.

I said that hearing voices isn't unusual and didn't mean he was going mad; that a small dose of sedatives from me, not the street, might help. And I asked him to come back tomorrow, to see one of the excellent mental health nurses, and to bring the name and number of his prison's social worker so that I might get in touch with them – which he did.

*

By 5 May the UK had again recorded the greatest number of deaths from Covid-19 in Europe – over 30,000. A week later the WHO was predicting the sharpest decline in the world economy since the 1930s depression – 3.2 per cent – and estimates were circulated that over 30 million people would be pushed into extreme poverty by the pandemic. Barack Obama made world headlines when he said of the current US administration that they 'aren't even pretending to be in charge'. UK unemployment almost tripled, from 800,000 to 2.1 million, and, as the number of worldwide confirmed cases passed 5 million, the Chinese government reported no new cases for the first time since January.

Through the nineteenth century the population of Edinburgh swelled as country folk moved in, either looking for the chance of a factory job or because they had been cleared from their own land to make way for sheep. Its overcrowding worsened, as did epidemics of disease. By the early 1860s the council appointed its first Medical Officer of Health: a man called Henry Littlejohn. At medical school, many of my tutorials took place in a suite of rooms that commemorate him; he established many of the measures that we now take for granted in safeguarding the health of the public.

Littlejohn was alarmed in particular by the death rate among infants from smallpox – at peaks it would cause the deaths of 10 per cent of all newborns. Given the effectiveness of inoculation, he lobbied from the beginning of his appointment for a new law demanding that all infants be vaccinated at six months of age. The authorities agreed, but didn't want to pay for it: from 1863 to 1867 parents were obliged get their children vaccinated but to fund it themselves. But four years was enough to prove the effectiveness of the programme, and then the town took over the cost. The will was there, the money was there, and the death rate from smallpox tumbled; it's been estimated that this single intervention saved over 100,000 lives.

Littlejohn was allocated two policemen who would patrol the city, vigilant for cases of infectious disease. They paid close attention to the fever hospitals and the lodging houses, just as in May 2020 contact tracing and disease control was concentrated around Covid clinics and homeless shelters. I'd heard from the charity volunteers at Streetwork how there had been complaints by some taxpayers as to how much funding and investment was going into helping the home-less population, but safeguarding public health has always required that kind of pragmatic compassion, spending money where it's needed to benefit not only the most vul-nerable but everyone else, too. It's just one of the debts that we owe to each other in society. In one nineteenth-century outbreak of smallpox at an Edinburgh lodging house Little-john persuaded everyone inside to get vaccinated by bribing them – at two shillings a head.

Just as every consultation about Covid-19 is coded on to a computer database, every death certificate has to detail whether the virus was a factor in that person's death. That, too, is a legacy of Littlejohn's innovations: from the late 1870s it was compulsory in Edinburgh for all doctors to notify the authorities if they saw anyone with scarlet fever, or smallpox, or typhus, or typhoid, or cholera, or diphtheria, or measles. For every case notified the doctor would be paid a couple of shillings; if it was found later that the doctor had failed to notify the authorities about a known case, a fine of forty shillings would be imposed. I heard that enquiries to Scot-land's death certification service had doubled since the start of the pandemic, as doctors sought advice for the dilemmas they faced in deciding whether to put 'Covid-19' as a factor on the death certificates they sent in when no positive swab had been recorded – particularly in the weeks before testing was widely available. Writing down 'coronavirus infection' as a factor in any death that happened in a care home would automatically subject that home to an investigation, and so there was immense pressure on both GPs and care home staff to make the certificates accurate, but also to reflect the uncertainty that is so much a part of good medical care.

The story of Edinburgh's Royal Infirmary is a powerful illustration of the ways in which epidemics and diseases have changed the urban landscapes we live in – and how, regardless of technological developments and modernity, as epidemics sweep back and forth across our communities, we find ourselves falling back on solutions which would not have seemed unfamiliar to people living centuries earlier. Each generation has its new treatments and technologies; and yet we are all starting with the same fallible human body, we are still at the mercy of new infections, and we are all too liable to forget what we have learned from the last.

During a major cholera epidemic in 1866, the Royal Infirmary filled up and refused to admit more patients, so the council set up a temporary infectious disease hospital in the city poorhouse – an old tenement in the Cowgate part of Edinburgh. (There was an echo of that situation in some London hospitals in March and April 2020, when oxygen – rather than beds – had become critically low and temporary overspill hospitals took up the excess admissions.) A few years later, the city's council made the arrangement permanent. This became Edinburgh's first 'fever hospital', just in time for a major smallpox epidemic in 1871. Ten years later, during an outbreak of scarlet fever, the infirmary was again overwhelmed and once more the 'fever hospital' threw open its doors.

In the 1880s the Royal Infirmary was relocated to its third iteration, a new build a few hundred yards away, and the City Fever Hospital, as it was called, took over the old eighteenth-century buildings at Infirmary Street. There were 260 beds available, isolation facilities for the most infectious patients, a quarantine ward for the families who'd been exposed to disease, and a disinfection unit for wiping down bedding and furniture from affected homes. The new hospital even had dedicated horse-and-cart ambulances – one for the exclusive use of scarlet fever patients, one for diphtheria patients, and one for those with typhoid fever. But when a simultaneous epidemic of smallpox and scarlet fever hit the city in 1894, even the City Fever Hospital couldn't cope – wooden huts were erected on Holyrood Park again, as they had been in the days of the medieval plagues. The city's population was pushing 300,000, and the squalor of Victorian industry was at its height. A new fever hospital was required, the third, and it was built to the south-west of the city beneath the hill of Craiglockhart. It had a capacity of 600 when it opened in 1903, and within a few years had expanded to 800 beds.

As a medical student in the 1990s I was taught here about virology and pandemic epidemiology. The city was then in recovery from the AIDS crisis, and new viral diseases were prominent in the minds of my tutors. I was told how the years of Littlejohn's tenure saw the city population double, while the death rate among infants fell by 20 per cent.* Littlejohn began his career in the years when miasma was thought to cause disease, and finished it in an age of universal vaccination and public sanitation. He oversaw the last cholera epidemic of the city in 1866, and was still alive for the last case of typhus in 1907.

---

* From 145 per 1,000 births to 114 per 1,000.

Until SARS-CoV-1, public health officials, epidemiologists and the World Health Organization had often assumed that the next great pandemic would, like Spanish flu or the 2009 swine flu, again be of influenza. That it turned out to be a coronavirus, the kind of virus that causes 5–10 per cent of common colds, took almost everyone by surprise. In retrospect, those public health tutorials were invaluable for learning about the hubris of medicine: more lives have been saved through better housing, sanitation and vaccination than were ever saved by a surgeon's knife or a physician's drugs.

By logging into the hospital computer system I kept an eye on Mr Magowan, read the ward round notes dictated by his consultant, looked at reports of the scans of his lungs, flicked through his laboratory results. He had pneumonia, and though his initial coronavirus swab came back negative, the specialists were suspicious, and were treating him as a case of Covid-19. His symptoms and deterioration were too characteristic of Covid-19 for it to be anything else, and their suspicions were confirmed on a subsequent swab. His wife wasn't allowed to visit. I felt for her, shielding herself at home and pacing around the otherwise empty house, waiting for news, the grandchildren's art on the walls and her hands fidgeting with her mobile phone, as she cleaned the house waiting, waiting for news.

One day, after my morning clinic had finished, I went down to the night shelter hotel in the city centre – separate from the hotel being looked after by Streetwork. At the entranceway there were signs in Polish, English and Romanian saying that if anyone was seen drinking alcohol they'd be asked to leave. At the makeshift reception desk, surrounded by cardboard boxes filled with brown paper food bags, I asked for Dr Budd. 'He'll in be in 217,' I was told, and was waved up one of the hotel staircases.

I've worked with John on and off for many years, crossing over with him often in the Edinburgh Access Practice, where he works full time. He has an air of unassailable calm, and a gentle, measured manner with patients that never shifts no matter the depth of the social or medical crisis he's called upon to help with (and I've called on him to advise and adjudicate in a few). I climbed the tartan-carpeted stairs, passing framed prints of twee Scottish scenes on every landing, and found him chatting with two junior doctors, Jennifer and Chantelle, both volunteers in the hotel clinics. Like the rest of their medical school year they had been obliged to qualify early, having had their final exams cancelled. John called their clinic work in the hotel 'Inclusion Health Outreach' – it was a way for them to help with the pandemic response before they took up their first jobs as junior doctors in August. John was about to go and see one of the patients they were worried about. 'Want to come along?' he asked me.

We climbed the stairs to another room to meet Martin. John knocked, and the door was opened by a bald, heavy-set man with a settled expression of rage on his face. There was a shiny scar from his forehead to his right eye, which caught the light of the fire exit signs. I looked down at the notes in my hand: he was the same age as me, but looked twenty years older. On the stairs John had told me he was just out of prison, where he'd been for eight years. *Eight years*, I thought, my mind skipping back over the events that had happened in my own life over those years, and how Martin had, for all that time, been caught in a web of institutional concrete.

In any normal summer in Edinburgh, the room would have been premium rate, with a view out over the Castle,

the Old Town and Princes Street Gardens. It was a beautiful summer afternoon and, in contrast to the electric buzz
and suppressed fury within, the city seemed a place of clean
order and harmony. In the room were stacks of food bank
tins, but nothing to heat them with; soup powder sachets
and instant noodles, too, and, in the corner, a hotel kettle.
The TV was on, loudly. John began talking to Martin about
his agitation and insomnia. 'It's all too much,' Martin said,
sweat shining on his scar. 'I can't even watch the telly, it's too
much.' John leaned to pick up the remote from where it lay
on the bed covers, and quietly switched off the sound. The
three of us stood there in silence for a few moments. 'Keep
things quiet, if that helps,' John said. 'And get out for long
walks, you can do that now.' He mentioned prescriptions,
support that was available, a counselling service that would
speak to Martin through a video link – he could get access to
a computer through the back of the hotel reception.

Out in the corridor, John told me it costs £40,000 a year
for someone to be kept in prison. 'So the state, having spent
£320,000 on him, has just turfed Martin out homeless, at
risk of violent reoffending, completely institutionalised.'
That Martin was unable to talk with anyone calmly, and was
unable to regulate his own reactions, was clear; it seemed
unfair he'd swapped a prison room for a hotel room, however
luxurious, condemned not to incarceration but to drinking
energy drinks and watching daytime television – imprisoned
not by the state, but by the pandemic. With employment
figures tumbling, he had little chance of finding any work,
and the kinds of anger management courses he needed
were all cancelled. 'Of course he's going out of his mind; of
course he can't sleep,' John said. 'I just hope he doesn't start
self-medicating.' Drug dealers had been hanging around at
the doors of the hotel. They'd been sent away, but of course
they'd be back.

There were a couple of other patients we visited, on the strangest 'ward round' I've ever been involved with, pacing the corridors of a luxury hotel. As we moved between the rooms I asked John Budd how many cases of coronavirus he'd had to deal with. 'We've been lucky so far,' he said. 'Just one! And we're better prepared now.' He laughed. 'This virus is like Voldemort – we know it's out there, and we know it's going to come back.'

By the end of May there had been just short of 40,000 Covid deaths in the UK. An American friend told me that in the US many doctors had been put out of work because their patients were staying away, afraid of infection and obeying their own local lockdowns, and there was no state support. 'Only in America', he said, 'would we be putting doctors out of work in a pandemic.'

Genetic studies of the virus were published: there were rumours that the virus in England came from China originally, and the one more prevalent in Scotland came from Iran and the Middle East. But that seemed counterintuitive, given the traffic between Scotland and England, and the number of cases that had come into the country from Italy in February. It was emerging that the virus was already being transmitted in Europe in the weeks before Christmas. 'In many countries,' a report in the *Guardian* concluded, 'including the UK, the variety of virus mutations sampled was almost as great as the variety seen across the whole world. This suggests the virus entered the UK lots of times independently, rather than via any one "patient zero" case that seeded the national epidemic.'

As I was cycling home in the rain, on one of the last days of the month, someone driving an orange Ford Fiesta almost killed me. The temperature was forecast to drop below freezing – the stunning run of sunny weather had ended. The city streets had been empty for so long that some drivers had begun to assume that emptiness complete, and were treating them as tunnels through which they could race unimpeded, rubber bouncing over cobbles. My mind was distracted that evening, slow, and that slowness in getting across the junction saved me: as the Fiesta accelerated into its red light, I swerved just in time, and the whistle of wet air as it passed me felt like an exhalation of relief. I was thankful, then, for the lumbering inertia I felt in my body and mind. The strap on my cycle helmet tugged at the hair on my cheeks; I realised it was a week or two since I'd shaved.

I'd been tired out by another day on the phone sifting through other people's anxieties, deciding which ones necessitated long conversations, which needed short conversations, who I would have to bring in to review face to face, or visor to visor, and who might need to see a psychiatrist. Part way through the day I'd logged into the hospital system and seen that Mr Magowan had died. 'I'll phone his wife tomorrow,' I thought – she'd be too upset to speak that day. And it was a relief to read in his notes that I hadn't lied about her being able to see him again: she had been allowed to visit him for the last day or two of his life.

On the way home I stopped off at the supermarket; the key worker at the till, a tall man with a West African accent, smiled and asked me how I had got so wet. I guessed most of his customers arrived from nearby stairwells, or carried umbrellas; they didn't turn up in rain-soaked waterproofs. I explained that I was part-way home, pedalling twelve miles, and that I always carry waterproof gear in my pannier for just such a May downpour as this. He smiled again. 'Good!' he said. 'After all, we live in Scotland!' and he seemed happy about that.

CONVALESCENCE

'[N]ow the people began to walk the streets again,
and those who were fled to return, there was no miss
of the usual throng of people in the streets ...'
Daniel Defoe
A Journal of the Plague Year

In the closing days of May the killing of George Floyd by a police officer in Minneapolis ignited protests against police brutality and institutional racism all over the world, including in Edinburgh. By the end of the first week in June, the protestors in England made headlines for toppling the prominent statue of a slave trader in Bristol, and for blocking a motorway in Warwickshire. The protestors in Edinburgh were asked to wear masks and keep two metres apart, but the Cabinet Secretary for Justice, Humza Yousaf, said that 'mass outdoor gatherings like this could present risk to public health ... we do know there is a lot of evidence of the disproportionate impact that Covid-19 can have on the minority ethnic community. So the very people whose lives we say matter are the very lives that those people could be putting at risk.'

I was sent an email from NHS Lothian detailing the board's commitment to equality, diversity and workplace safety: 'As we move forward, it will be more important than ever to address the inequalities in society and in our organisation which lead to unequal health outcomes, and be part of the movement to end racism.'

In response to specific questions raised by the BAME network of NHS Lothian staff they promised to:

1. Support all managers to proactively identify and talk with BME staff to have supportive conversations and offer appropriate risk assessments.
2. Work with partnership, other Boards, and Scottish Government, to ensure we contribute to and adopt a Risk Assessment that explicitly acknowledges and reflects ethnicity and its impact on risk.
3. Ensure that as evidence continues to clarify, we are better prepared for any second wave of Coronavirus infection, and able to proactively support and protect as necessary any and all our staff who may be at increased risk.
4. Develop our Race Equality Action Plan in partnership with the BME Staff Network.
5. Ensure executive leadership attendance at the next BME staff network.

There was an algorithm for staff members to follow to figure out whether they might be at increased or decreased risk from the virus. There was still very little known about the reason for worse Covid-19 outcomes among black and south Asian people in the UK. A connection with low vitamin D levels had been proposed. An April review in *The Lancet* had asked whether BAME communities might be at increased risk because of higher levels of diabetes, high blood pressure and heart disease, but also asked whether ethnicity 'could interplay with virus spread through cultural, behavioural, and societal differences including lower socioeconomic status, health-seeking behaviour, and intergenerational cohabitation'. Two months later, another *Lancet* review was unable to elaborate further. 'The lack of association between ethnicity and COVID-19 mortality after adjustment for comorbidities is not reassuring,' it concluded. 'This suggests that research into ethnic disparities in COVID-19 mortality must consider social as well as biological factors.' Many of my colleagues with south Asian parentage were mystified, and anxious about their own risk – but continued to work on the front line against the virus.

The message said only 'mood – to discuss', and the appointment was made by the girl's grandmother, whom I knew well. I took a look through the notes, and saw nothing else to go on. I'd seen her six years earlier for an ear infection, a couple of years earlier than that following a gymnastics injury, but beyond that there were only vaccinations and a few entries from the toddler years. I couldn't picture her face but, with the passage of six years and the transformations of puberty, she might be beyond recognition anyway. Unusually for a 16-year-old I had been given a mobile phone number: it rang but no one picked up, and there was no way to leave a message. I tried the land line of the house, but no one answered that either. Odd, in lockdown, to be unable to get anyone to answer the phone. I left as neutral a message as I thought I could get away with, and hung up.

It was later in the morning that Stella called back. I introduced myself, and thanked her for ringing. 'What would you like to talk about?' I asked.

Her voice seemed very small, uncertain, but at the same time there was bravery in it. 'Dunno, I guess the way I've been feeling?'

'And how's that?'

'Just low, really low,' she said. 'Panicky, worried.'

'Mm. Anything else?'

'And what's next, I think, I can't see …' Her voice tailed off. 'I can't see how all this is going to end.'

'All what?'

'I can't imagine when I'll be able to see my friends.'

'How have you been managing with lockdown, what have you been doing?'

'Nothing much.'

There was a silence and I tried to resist the temptation to fill the space with talk. After a few seconds she spoke again. 'I read novels. SF novels.'

'Do you get out? You know you can go out every day for some exercise,' I said.

'I sometimes walk the dog,' she said.

I made a noise which I hoped would convey agreement, understanding, support, affirmation, while avoiding censure. As in: 'You should go out more.' I imagined she was hearing that kind of thing already, from her parents and from her grandmother.

'You said you get really low, or panicky,' I said. 'Is that a new thing?'

There was another silence, and I felt the oddness of the space between us, the electric wires bridging the distance between our voices but doing nothing to bridge the gap between the teenage and the middle-aged, the roles allocated to both of us, and which we were both trying to see past. Her suffering and my attempted understanding, her youth and my experience, both of having been through a nervous adolescence myself and having spoken with so many anguished teenagers over twenty years of clinical practice. I wondered whether I was helping at all, or was I just another ageing fool pretending he could empathise?

'No,' she said at last. 'It's not a new thing.'

'And what did you used to do before Covid, before the pandemic, when you felt like this?'

I could *hear* her shrug. 'I used to bite my lip a bit, or the inside of my cheek,' she said. 'Until it passed.'

'And now?'

She took a deep breath. 'At the beginning I was scratching myself, with nail clippers.'

'And now?' I repeated.

'I haven't done that for a while,' she said.

'That's good.' I waited a few moments to see if she'd say anything else, but she didn't. 'Lots of people find that when they're feeling really upset, making themselves hurt is a way of clearing their mind, or making things feel more real,' I said. 'But it's not a good idea – there are other, better ways of coping with those feelings. Have you got scars?'

'Some.'

'Where?'

'On my ankle. I figured they'd be less obvious there.'

'Have you heard of other ways of dealing with those kinds of feelings? Anything else you've tried?'

'No.'

'I can send you some ideas for other things to do; to distract yourself, I mean.'

'Ok then.' There was another silence for a few moments.

'Who else is at home?' I asked.

'My mum and dad, my big brother.'

'And can you talk to any of them? Tell them how you've been feeling?'

'No.'

'What about friends?'

'Some …' I heard her voice catch with tears. 'My boyfriend. But I haven't, haven't' – her voice cracked – 'I haven't seen him since … before all this.'

So much of the support and welfare of teenagers is conducted through schools, it seemed suddenly extraordinary to me that schooling had simply been cancelled overnight;

that consideration hadn't been given to keeping channels of communication open for pupils to be in touch with teachers that offer support. I'd asked a neighbour who works as a high school teacher how he was coping with seeing his pupils only by video, as we in general practice were having to do, and I was surprised when he shook his head. 'No videos allowed,' he said. 'These kids are in their bedrooms, and we can't be looking into their bedrooms. It's as much to protect me as to protect them.' But this policy brought in to protect vulnerable children and adolescents had deepened the catastrophic isolation being endured by so many of them. I wondered how difficult it would have been for local authorities to get some kind of disclaimer or permission form for parents, so that teachers could stay in contact more visibly with their pupils.

'I don't think that will be for much longer,' I said to Stella. 'Things are easing up soon. You'll be able to see your boyfriend, I'm sure.'

'I can't see how anything is ever going to get back to normal,' she said.

I caught an image, suddenly, from her perspective, of her inability to see any future, any possibility of one day having the freedom to walk somewhere hand in hand with her boyfriend, to study at college, to party, to dance; it all seemed suddenly unreal to her, as if, in the insulating cushion of protectiveness being forced around her, she was forgetting how to feel.

'It'll get better, I'm sure of it,' I said. 'Things will get better for you.' I hesitated for a moment, wondering if the line I was taking was helping, or making things worse. 'It's no fun being sixteen at the best of times,' I said. 'And being sixteen in the middle of a global pandemic must be terrible.' I waited a minute, but it seemed as if she wanted me to go on. 'On one level it's good that you're getting this all over with now – with luck we'll be free of this virus by the time you're eighteen.' That got a small laugh – a triumph.

As we spoke on the telephone I was checking out the website of a local mental health charity for teens – only to see that it too was closed, because of the pandemic. Why it had closed when the majority of its counselling work had always been over the telephone I had no idea, but it was another example of how the gains made over the past few years in prioritising mental health as much as physical health had been forced into reverse by the virus.

'I've got some things I'd like to send you,' I said. 'About anxiety, about alternatives to scratching yourself, about how to find the right way for you to calm yourself and help you get through this. Should I post it or email it or would you like to come and collect it?'

'I could collect it.'

'And if you're down here anyway, do you prefer that we just check in like this on the phone every week, or do you want to come in and chat to me face to face.'

'Come in,' she said, without hesitation.

We GPs were still being discouraged from holding face to face consultations – they were only for emergencies, we were told, or for ruling out dangerous diagnoses such as cancer. But seeing a teenager in crisis seemed as valid a reason as any. Though the counselling of people who scratch themselves is not, I admit, my specialist area, I felt glad to be able to restore to my daily work one of its fundamental principles: to *see* people in distress, and make an attempt, if not at healing, then at listening and trying to understand. To confront face to face the undifferentiated unhappiness that has always been the core of a GP's work, rather than trying to do it all down a telephone line.

The whole country was waiting, waiting for this nightmare to pass. Talking with Stella reminded me of a line in

Tom Robbins' novel *Even Cowgirls Get The Blues*, about the damage of perpetual waiting: 'workers who can't be happy until they've retired, adolescents who can't be happy until they've grown, ill people who can't be happy until they're well ... and, in most cases, vice versa, people waiting, waiting for the world to begin'.

In just three months I'd been involved in detaining under the Mental Health Act ('sectioning') two of my psychiatric patients for their own good – a high rate for General Practice, where once every couple of years is more common. These occasions are always difficult, and had been made ten times more so by the fact that I, the psychiatrist, the mental health officer and even the police were all in masks and gloves – not a good look when going to meet someone suffering from paranoid psychosis. In a conversation with a psychiatrist friend I heard of a spike in psychosis up and down the country in people with no history of it before. Coronavirus *per se* was not responsible for this surge in psychotic breakdowns, but the extraordinary circumstances into which we'd all been pushed were. The lockdown was revealing all kinds of vulnerabilities, in-born as well as stress-induced, that hitherto had remained hidden. It struck me again forcefully that this was a health crisis whose implications stretched far beyond the confines of ITUs and infected lungs – it was touching almost every aspect of my patients' lives.

At a Lothian-wide medical meeting online, Dr Andrew Watson, one of the city psychiatrists, detailed the startling number of new cases of psychosis he was seeing, including one patient who believed he was on a mission from God to rid the world of coronavirus and another who since the death of George Floyd had become withdrawn, paranoid, despairing. 'Many are middle-aged,' he said, 'and male, with no psychiatric history at all.' He wondered at the mix of triggers: changing patterns of substance abuse and alcohol, the loss of the usual coping strategies that we all evolve to deal with distress, amputation from networks of social support, distance from extended family, financial calamity, the cabin fever of being stuck at home. I wondered if there was something about masculinity, too, and traditional male social roles. As society was being drastically restructured, changes to routine could be a trigger for many, and also that stresses that once found an outlet beyond the home were now being revealed through confinement – imprisonment – within it. Wellbeing ratings for happiness, anxiety and life satisfaction were all worsening, particularly for women, and Watson wondered how much our national anxiety was feeding into the psychosis: 'The world can become pregnant with meaning,' he said. 'Everything seems different, and what was important no longer seems so.' This societal change might, Watson hoped, even offer us insights into what it's like to develop psychotic illness. 'Perhaps,' he concluded hopefully, 'a positive outcome will be a greater sense that we are all in it together, people with severe mental illness included.'

It was the middle of June, and the children had now been out of school for three months. Some non-essential goods shops had begun to open with restrictions, as well as outdoor venues such as zoos, but in England only children in Early Years and Years 1 and 6 had been allowed to return to school. Across the UK there was a growing disquiet about the consequences for children, and a friend of mine got in touch to ask if I'd join her and others in writing to the Scottish education secretary, John Swinney.

Becky Sutherland is one of the consultant physicians in Edinburgh's Infectious Diseases unit. We were at medical

school together, where she was a star student, and her dili-
gence has never let up. After qualifying from Edinburgh she
went to Oxford to train jointly in microbiology and infectious diseases, and then set up HIV clinics in rural southern
Africa. She's smart and dedicated, composed and wry, with a
droll sense of humour that pops up at unexpected moments.

Back in February Becky saw the first Covid-19 patient
in Lothian. I knew she'd hardly had a day off since. She
introduced me to a group of physicians, GPs, nurses and paediatricians by email, and together we drafted a letter:

Dear Mr Swinney,
I am writing to ask if your team would reconsider the
severity of restrictions placed on schools in Scotland.

We are a group of Infectious Disease physicians and
nurses, Paediatricians and General Practitioners who
have worked at the front line of the Covid-19 pandemic
since February.

We understand the concern around disease transmission in schools and the desire to protect both staff
and pupils from Covid-19 disease. We are aware of how
much work schools are putting in to make the environment as safe as possible and the challenge this poses.
However, we feel that the health and social well-being
benefits of access to school for children far outweigh any
risks to children individually. It is of course essential that
risk mitigating strategies are employed to reduce any
risk as far as possible to adults working within schools.

We are aware of the effort employed to enable the
NHS in Scotland to manage this pandemic, including
the construction of a new NHS hospital in Glasgow
in an astonishingly short amount of time. We ask that
the same priority and collective action is now taken to
ensure a generation of children do not miss out on vitally

important schooling, further entrenching inequality in society and allowing the most vulnerable children in our communities to carry the greatest burden.

It should be specifically noted that throughout the pandemic in Edinburgh, of approximately 50,000 school age children, only 15 have so far tested positive for SARS-CoV-2, and very few have required hospital admission. 2725 tests have been carried out in individuals less than 17 years and there have been no positive tests in children since the 4th of April. This should provide some reassurance.

Children have carried a heavy burden for society over the past few months without compelling evidence that they pose a risk to others. We feel that their continued mental and physical health needs are very important and will be further compromised by the lack of access to schooling.

We feel that the government has acted to mitigate a measurable harm (Covid-19 deaths among adults) by perpetrating innumerable less measurable harms on those in our communities with the least autonomy, and the least to fear from the virus. It is time that we confront this small risk head on with a pragmatic approach, not one based on fear and hearsay.

Signed ...

It was one letter among hundreds that government officials across the UK were receiving – two days later, on 17 June, over 1,500 paediatricians wrote to the UK Prime Minister with the same demand.

Perhaps the summative effect of all those letters was to make a contribution to government policy, or perhaps ministers were confirmed in their decisions long before they were received, but shortly afterwards it was announced that schools in Scotland would return on 12 August, without social distancing measures.

There was a day in June when I spoke with three people aged 88, and two aged 91, one of whom I visited shortly afterwards. She had been a shop owner in the Lake District for most of her life, but had washed up in Edinburgh – the city of her birth – after decades of the usual dramas: illnesses, dependency, her husband's needs and his dwindling autonomy. A tall woman, proud, with a pharaonic nose and a chimney brush of hair that she inexpertly dyed, she used to come and see me in the clinic in a floral dress and hiking boots. I enjoyed her visits.

To get into her flat now I have to punch a code into the kind of keysafe used for holiday lets, and keep the keys from her once I'm in – she is to be a prisoner in her own home now, for her own safety, though the week before she was found in the garden in her nightdress, reluctant to be led back inside. It had been months now since I'd seen her on her feet – and weeks since she had even had the television on as I came in.

Often on my visits I get the keys from the keysafe, call theatrically from the door, only to find her dozing in a chair. She wakes with a start at a gentle hand on her shoulder – she doesn't hear very well, and I have to speak up. The usual formalities are dispensed with now, we know one another too well, and she begins by commenting on my ridiculous attire – the plastic apron and the gloves, the mask that makes it almost impossible for people like her, the hard of hearing, to appreciate what I am saying. I compromise and, sitting two metres back from her, pull it down so that she can at least see my lips move.

Before the pandemic broke she was on the cusp of being

admitted to a care home. Because of it we'd had to put those plans on hold. But the issue evolving in June was how much longer could we go on waiting? Four months in, it was clear that restrictions would go on into 2021 – and that the winter was as likely to bring another surge as an improvement. I would have to find somewhere for her to be safe, where she wouldn't fall, where she'd have human company.

She had worsening breathlessness, and I wondered if there was a cancer in her lungs. Her breath caught when I asked her to breathe in for the stethoscope, the almost century-old skin of her chest creased and pliable, no elasticity left in it. I murmured about tests, about scans, mentioned the word cancer – the first time warily, watching her expression, and the second time with more confidence, after establishing that, as for the majority of nonagenarians, the word holds no fear for her. And no, she didn't want me to send her for any tests.

I was worried, too, about her memory, which seemed to be deteriorating, and established that, although she knew the year and the month and the day, she had no idea where she was now living. When I gave her prompts, she told me about the factory that stood on the site of her housing block seventy years ago, and how she'd passed it often as a young woman. And then, apropos of nothing other than the sense she felt somewhere within her that I was testing her memory, she began a long story about being bullied by her brother, punched in the gut, in the head, thrown across the room. 'I was never the same since,' she said.

'How old were you?' I ask.

'Six or seven,' she replied, and I realised that she had been dwelling on the memory of this incident for decades, and for nearly ninety years had wondered whether there was something deeply wrong with her, some silent injury and fear of perpetual damage that she had been nursing long after that brother had forgotten what he did. 'He's dead now', she added, then repeated the story of having been held and punched. I did a quick calculation – this must have happened in about 1936.

As she told me the story, her one good eye moving away from mine and drifting towards the cornicing of the room, I saw that the incident was so much more real to her than I was, so much more vivid than this room, this lockdown lonely life.

Later I called her nephew, and told him that I wouldn't be referring his aunt to have her cough investigated, and that I thought we should go ahead and make arrangements for her to go into the care home, despite all the restrictions of the pandemic. She had already detached herself from this world, and any resistance that she showed now to the idea was little more than inertia, ballast, and that it was up to us now to make use of tiller and tide.

Towards the end of June I left the Forth estuary for Orkney in the heavy fog known locally as 'haar' – a linguistic legacy of Norse rule – through clouds brought to earth. The record-breaking sunshine through April and May had very much come to an end. 'Ye'll have had your summer,' as they say in Scotland. And driving north through the glens of the High-land Line, along empty highways, I spotted scattered rainbow commemorations thanking NHS workers, each triggering a spasm of guilt in me – there was little Covid in evidence now, and I didn't feel I was putting myself very much at risk. Twenty health and social care workers in Scotland had died of the virus, although UK-wide that figure had passed 600. Though the seismic wash of it had swept away so much of the way I used to work, those thank you rainbows felt unjustified for me personally, and even though the risk remained, the gratitude felt unearned. At least the Thursday claps had stopped.

Through the high granite heart of Scotland the sky cleared and I drove in sunshine, winding down the windows to cool off as the car ticked off the passes with gutteral, earth-laden names: Birnam, Drumochter, Slochd. In the supermarket I stopped off at in Inverness there were more masks in evidence than further south, and I slid beneath the stylite of the hospital chimney, glad to be heading on further north where the road sidles to the strandline: Tain, Dornoch, Golspie, Helmsdale. The legacy of Scandinavians is written on the roadsigns of eastern Scotland, dotted between the now-familiar illuminated signs still reading 'STAY HOME, PROTECT THE NHS, SAVE LIVES'.

In Golspie an old man was collecting rubbish, humming to himself, and the car park by the beach, ordinarily full at this time of year, was haunted instead by hungry-looking crows. The tide was out. I lay on the sand and snoozed for half an hour in the sunshine. On the eastern horizon, out over the North Sea, there was the same grey barrier of haar that I'd left behind in Lothian.

Thurso is dubbed Scotland's 'Atomic City' for its proximity to and subsistence from the nuclear reactor of Dounreay, and it's reached through a boulevard of wind turbines. They're ice white and otherworldly, wheeling over the featureless moor, each blade a delicate wing of aerodynamic perfection. In the port of Scrabster, where the Orkney ferry leaves, there was sun, wind and fulmars playing over the updrafts from the cliffs. The ferry office was locked, but illuminated notices proclaimed that 'Non-essential travel to the Northern Isles will be Refused'. After half an hour a car pulled up, and two women in navy fleeces branded for the ferry company got out and unlocked the office. It took them ten minutes to switch on all the lights, pull up the blinds, crank up their computers and pull back the window, leaving an absurdly short perspex screen between them and me, which certainly wouldn't protect them from my coughs or sneezes. They discussed my letter from Orkney Health Board confirming that I was an essential worker, asked to see my driving licence, and then typed up a government form querying my purpose in visiting Orkney. 'So, you're an Edinburgh doctor going to work where – in the hospital?'

'I'm going to work at the Covid Assessment Centre,' I said.

She mouthed it out as she typed.

'One way?'

'No, I'll be back in a week.'

There were just three other cars waiting for the ferry built to take sixty-eight – I wondered idly if the other drivers were working for the gas, electricity and water boards. It seemed almost absurd to pay for a ticket at all, given that no one was allowed on board unless they were fulfilling an essential service – Scottish ferries are government-subsidised to the tune of £200 million per year. An eerie absence had settled over the ferry's walkways, eateries, lounges, shops, amusement arcades – all closed off.

The west mainland of Orkney is a shallow bowl of light, edged with cliffs of red sandstone. Two lochs lie in its saucer – one of freshwater and one of salt. From above they look like hinged wings, or the chambers of a heart. Leaving the harbour of Stromness, I drove east through dregs of fog to Kirkwall. It had been a long drive north; I found my billet near the hospital, and slept.

The Covid Assessment Centres had been set up urgently in March, all over the country, to keep coronavirus patients away from their usual GPs' surgeries. In Edinburgh an evening and weekend centre had had to close to make room for one, but in Orkney they were fortunate to have an old hospital awaiting demolition. I'd worked in that hospital between ten and fourteen years before, and it was sad to see it look so abandoned. Some of the wire barriers had been taken down and a wing had been opened up again for use. I locked up my bike, which I'd brought with me, and sat down on the grass to wait. At 8 a.m. a car pulled up, a hand waving out of its window.

Anne had been working in Orkney's Covid Assessment Centre since it began. She led me through to an old reception space and introduced me to Angela, the manager – a nurse by training, she told me her daughter works in an ITU in London, and she knew just how lightly they'd had it in Orkney. Of the rest of the team, most had had nothing to do with healthcare before the pandemic. Of the drivers who brought in patients with cough and fever for testing, one was a jeweller, another a plumber, and another a student who had been sent home from his campus. The cleaning staff had arrived en masse when the bar and restaurant at which they had worked closed back in March. The swabbing team, who were testing all the residents of the island's care homes in rotation, were all on furlough from dental practices.

Protocols, crib sheets, proformas, checklists: it was comforting to me that wherever you practise medicine its bureaucracy remains the same. And the virus, too: many of the precautions I was being asked to carry out here were familiar to me from my work in Edinburgh.

There's a phone call: a GP colleague is just back from a visit to a care home. An old woman is coughing, short of breath, and he asks if I'll come out and perform the swab to check if it's Covid.

The 'doctor's' car is awaiting a mechanic, but I'm tossed the keys of another, and soon afterwards I'm driving beneath a hot summer sky, fields golden with buttercups; Radio Orkney is playing on the car stereo, reporting on the latest scandal in the council, the crisis in the islands' tourism, a centenarian's birthday celebration. Covid has turned care homes in Edinburgh into prisons, large 'NO VISITORS' signs are routine, and all across the country residents and staff are now regularly swabbed to prevent the kinds of care home outbreaks that proved so devastating in April and May. In Orkney the visiting of care homes is suspended, too, but the front doors are wide open when I arrive and I'm met not by a poster listing risks but one in rainbow lettering which reads 'You don't live where we work, we work in your home'. It's a sentiment that, in the rising panic over outbreaks in nursing homes, has been all too often forgotten by journalists: even with the terrible risk, to turn care homes into sterile fortresses would be a dismal and retrograde step.

I've a box of PPE under one arm, and on the threshold I put it down and begin the palaver. In Orkney they have disposable gowns of thin blue plastic instead of aprons, and I put my arms through the sleeves, then snap on my gloves over the cuffs. Visors are disposable here and, if not attending a cardiac resuscitation, we are not required to wear a tight, face-fitting mask. With my blue plastic gown rustling over my peach surgical scrubs, I hope I don't encounter any residents in the corridor while looking for someone to take me to the patient. A couple of shouted 'Hello's' and a head appears around a doorway, smiling a welcome, and I think: Yes, this is a good care home. Smiling staff and happy residents.

My patient is bed bound and sits propped up on pillows, while a young man with an apron over a rock band T-shirt and wearing DIY goggles is helping her swallow a syrup of antibiotics. His voice is tender, encouraging – back in the base I'd mentioned the name of the patient I was going to swab, and immediately there were nods of recognition. In this community the people might be strung out across the landscape , but their connections are denser than in the city, perhaps even as a consequence of that space – and they are often stronger, too. The carer knows her well, and holds her hand as I explain what I'm there to do.

I know her dementia is advanced, she has pneumonia, that my accent will seem odd to her, and my appearance here in plastic sheeting, mask and visor will, for her, have the character of a fever dream rather than of a reasoned conversation. 'You've a chest infection,' I say to her. She nods. 'And we need to know what's causing that infection.' I hold up the swab – a cotton bud on a stalk of plastic: 'I've to put this at your throat and your nose, to see what's causing your trouble.' She nods again.

Obliging me, she opens her mouth, but when the swab hits the soft palate of her throat she gags, bites down and tries to hit my hand away. I try to circle it there, appreciating her discomfort, for the required ten seconds, and pull it out just before she bites down.

'Your nose, too,' I say, and almost incredibly, she nods again. The swab goes back, and back, and back – 'This feels a bit strange,' I hear myself say – and there, too, I tickle it on the membranes at the centre of her head for a further ten seconds.

Then it's out into the corridor, pulling at the blue plastic gown that clings to the sweat on my forearms. I yank it off and stuff it into an orange clinical waste bag, along with the top layer of gloves and visor, and begin to clean the surface of my box. On a bench in the care home lobby, sitting in the sunshine, one of the residents is playing the accordion. I struggle a moment to place the tune: Louis Armstrong's 'What a Wonderful World'.

'There's a baby at the hub.' I receive a text message while I am down in the town, getting something to eat. I'd changed out of my pastel peach scrubs, so as not to give too odd an impression walking around town, and was sitting at the pier head in the sun, thinking about how rare it is in Orkney that the sun feels warm enough for discomfort. 'I'll be there in five minutes,' I said.

For any doctor on call for emergencies, advance notice of an unwell baby provokes a mixture of emotions: anxiety or dread are prominent, because small babies can be so difficult to assess, and can become critically ill so rapidly. But often for me there's a curiosity, too: before babies learn to focus or to smile they seem to live in a kind of borderland, no longer beings of the womb but not yet fully of our world. This baby has a fever, I'm told – 39.5 – and isn't feeding properly. Though it's vanishingly unlikely that the baby has Covid-19, all fevered children are to be assessed in the Covid Assessment Centre to rule out the virus.

Her mother is Polish, I think, or maybe Latvian, and wears a flowered scarf pulled up around her nose. 'I've had the virus,' she tells me when she sees my mask and visor. 'I had it back in March, when I was pregnant.'

'Here?' I ask her.

'London.'

The baby is in a sling, asleep, her face pushed into her mother's breast. It's impossible, as ever, to imagine her wailing until she starts. I watch the flicker of her pulse over the soft spot on the top of her head, the spot that allowed the plates of her skull to flex and overlap during birth. Her temperature is 38 now, after medication, and her breaths are short and rapid, clean and full of life. Her mum peels her from the sling and her eyes open briefly. They swim towards mine, milky and opaque, but pass on to something more interesting: the contrast my ear makes against the light falling in from the window, perhaps. As I watch her, I think of the millions upon millions of connections whistling their codes to one another through her developing brain, how with each breath, and each reaching out to the world, millions are in retreat while millions more are being reinforced. 'She has these lumps,' says her mother. 'What's wrong with her?'

'What lumps?'

Her fingertips trace a low topography over the back of her daughter's skull, an upturned V-shaped ridge with a tail, like the Greek letter λ. There is fear in the mother's eyes, and I rush, perhaps too quickly, to diffuse it.

'Don't worry,' I said, 'that's just the skull bones, settling into place after birth.'

The mother looked downcast instead of relieved. 'I'm so sorry to bother you,' she said, 'in the middle of ...' With a shrug she indicates the whole pandemic. ' ... in the middle of all this.'

'That's what I'm here for,' I said, wishing I could have more of these kinds of consultations, more problems with easy answers, simple resolutions, rather than virus, virus, virus.

Despite my fears in February, the people of Orkney had been protected from the virus – there had been only a handful of cases. In the week I worked at the assessment centre only one swab came back positive – and the patient was swiftly quarantined. The islanders' natural isolation had protected them, though the fear of it, in comparison with in the cities further south, was more pronounced. I heard that on the island of Westray anyone who had been to Kirkwall was asked to stay away from the village shop for a fortnight. There was fury at a health board executive who worked in Orkney but whose home was a hundred miles or so further south – his weekly commutes were felt to have put all the islanders at risk. Pavements were near empty in Kirkwall, but pedestrians would still cross to the other side of the street to avoid sharing space. All to the good, I thought; their caution was working well for them so far.

The sacrifices made by those healthcare teams I'd worked with in February were extreme: island doctors were self-isolating for a fortnight or more before arriving to take up their posts, to ensure there would be no risk of their carrying the virus into the small communities that had seen no cases. Other doctors and nurses who were ordinarily based further south had stayed in Orkney throughout the pandemic, passing month after month there, not seeing their families, so as to protect their patients. A trio of Westray doctors hadn't been off the island at all. At the Covid hub Angela had been replaced by Karen, the nurse I'd worked with back in February. She filled me in on how all the patients we'd seen together then were faring, and she spoke with a typical islander's nonchalance of the difficulties and triumphs of setting up a Covid service for the archipelago.

The weather was the kind that makes city-dwellers want to relocate north. For my last night in Kirkwall, 21 June, the harbour water was the stillest I'd ever seen it, a smooth pool of gold in the solstice sunlight at 10 p.m., unimaginable that it could be the same bay I saw churning through those storms in February. As I watched the water, my thoughts alternated between a kind of blank acceptance of the changes the pandemic had forced on to all of our lives, and a sweaty horror at the depth of the shock to society, the difficulties and miseries that had been ignited by it.

The following day I sailed south, back to my Edinburgh practice. A minke whale surfaced briefly off the starboard side of the ferry; there were shearwater fly-pasts, fulmars and puffins. As we approached the coast of Caithness the black wing tips of a gannet flashed in the distance, like a cursor blinking on the blank screen of the sky.

It was the end of June, and there were – at last – short runs of days in which no one in Scotland died of Covid-19. The first results of the RECOVERY Trial were published: of all the drugs and interventions being researched it was one of the oldest, the steroid dexamethasone, that was proven to be of the most benefit to those with life-threatening Covid-19. Overnight, worldwide hospital-based protocols of treatment changed, with every patient that might benefit from it being given the drug. It was a relief that it was one of the cheapest and most widely available of the medicines tested that had proven to be most effective.

On Friday 26 June in Glasgow, a man from Sudan living in a city centre hotel being used by the Home Office to house evicted asylum seekers, stabbed six other people, including a police officer, before being shot by Special Forces. It was said that he was suffering from a paranoid psychosis. Some of the men in the hotel had been sharing rooms, and concerns had apparently been raised about the dead man's mental health.

I heard that fasting through Ramadan had been difficult or even impossible for Muslim residents of the hotel-turned-detention centre because canteen food was provided only at routine mealtimes – breakfast, lunch and dinner. Some had lost contact with friends and family. The lockdown had imposed extraordinary stresses on the residents and, as Andrew Watson had already pointed out, Covid-19 was bringing out severe distress in many people who had never before had issues with mental health. And, as I'd seen in my conversations with Stella, being inside for week after week, with no hope of lockdown lifting, and little autonomy, could ignite the most intense anguish among the stable and well supported, leading to the kind of deliberate self-harm that she used as a coping strategy.

Yet the figures for the medical benefits of lockdown were incontrovertible: at the end of June, deaths in Scotland were down to single figures each week and new cases per day were at less than twenty nationwide. Though as the pandemic dwindled in my own country, it accelerated elsewhere: 28 June saw the global death toll pass 500,000, with the number of proven cases at 10 million.

Both case numbers and Covid deaths continued to drop across Europe, though outbreaks associated with food factories, abattoirs and meat-packing plants flared in both the UK and Germany, showing how the virus can thrive in closed, air-conditioned spaces with refrigeration and a lack of natural light. By the last week in June, the 'excess deaths' figures released by the National Records office showed that, with respect to its death rate, Scotland was back to normal – the same number of people died that week as had died in comparable weeks of earlier years. The whole of June had felt like a convalescence under way – exhausting, slow, but welcome, a stretching back into the light. That light was illuminating scars across the whole of society, inflicted by the first wave of the virus. Such a brief period, but it was already clear that they would take years or even decades to heal.

RESPITE

*'The physicians opposed this thoughtless humour of the people
with all their might ... advising the people to continue reserved,
and to use still the utmost caution in their ordinary conduct ...'*
Daniel Defoe
A Journal of the Plague Year

In my late twenties I worked as the medical officer at the
most isolated research station operated by the British government, on the Brunt Ice Shelf in Antarctica. The base was
a few hundred miles from the South Pole, where the ozone
hole, meteorology and solar wind were tracked and studied
by scientists. There were just fourteen of us for the year, and
for ten months of that year the sea was frozen for hundreds
of miles around us; we were unreachable by ship or by plane.
It was for my role there that I had taken my Diploma in the
Medical Care of Catastrophes which had seemed so terrify-
ingly relevant in March.

The SARS-CoV-1 pandemic occurred while I was
deployed in Antarctica. My colleagues – all scientists and
tradesmen – were relatively young, fit and healthy, and we
lived in a quarantine world of silence, ice and light. There
was a dial-up satellite modem that brought news by text-only
email once a day, but otherwise we were isolated in a pristine,
sterile world – news of the pandemic felt utterly irrelevant.

After a year of that separation from society the first plane to land was from a German polar expedition. It stopped at our base to refuel, on its way to another station a few hundred miles to our east. It brought a crate of fresh fruit from Latin America – glorious tastes, almost forgotten smells! – and a couple of days after it left us, we all came down with a common cold.

In July, I once again found myself connected to this period of my life: after I'd finished my afternoon clinics, I had half-hour appointments to conduct medical examinations on a series of scientists and tradespeople who were about to be deployed to Antarctica. Ordinarily these are conducted in Cambridge, where the British Antarctic Survey (BAS) has its headquarters, or in Plymouth, where the Medical Unit of BAS is based, but pandemic travel restrictions meant that former BAS doctors had been asked if they could carry out the medicals closer to applicants' homes. There are places in Antarctica from which medical evacuation is impossible for much of the year, and so over five weeks I assessed plumbers, electricians, divers, mountaineers, both in terms of their general fitness and to gauge the likelihood of their becoming ill once deployed.

The speed with which the virus flourished through cruise ship populations shows just how dangerous it can be in closed settings, far from land. Most of these Antarctic personnel would sail there by ship as I had, in a journey that takes between two and three months. I heard grim stories of people being cooped up in hotel rooms in the Falkland Islands for two weeks straight, and everyone I assessed would be obliged to self-isolate for two weeks before boarding the ship that would take them south. 'I'm jealous,' I joked with them, as one by one they came from all corners of Scotland to be assessed at my clinic. 'It's not such a bad idea to sit out this pandemic on the ice.' By the time they came home it would be 2022. Surely we'd have the virus under control by then?

Increasingly as the lockdown eased and infection rates fell, we were offered a tantalising glimpse of a return to the pre-pandemic world, and wondered how long that shift towards reopening could be sustained. A space began to open up in which it was possible to reckon with what we'd been through and, encouraged by news of the multiple vaccines now entering clinical trials, think about how we might ever find a way back to the 'old normal'. Some of my patients were still shielding from the virus, and though people had been encouraged to return to their workplaces, society as a whole felt very much wrapped in restrictions and Covid-secure rules. We knew more about how to treat the disease in its damaging immunological phase, but the virus remained as dangerous, and transmissible, as ever. There was, as yet, no end in sight.

Humanity's co-evolution with viruses has been useful, even essential – we all carry reams of viral DNA in our genetic signatures, embedded there millennia ago, and it's been proposed that the ability of viruses to interfere with our genetic code has even helped our evolution by facilitating mutations. Each of us is assailed by myriad viruses every day and, for the most part, we get rid of them thanks to the agility of our immune systems. Much of this is due to antibodies: long, complex proteins free-floating in our bloodstream and expressed on the surfaces of our nose, lungs, and guts. They bind to any proteins recognised as being 'foreign', whether viral or bacterial, then clump together to neutralise the threat. Other elements of the immune system recognise when a body cell has become infected (one lining the lungs, say, or the intestine) and sacrifice it before it can build copies of the virus.

Yet the system isn't foolproof, or infectious disease would

be unknown: there are frequent mismatches, and many germs and viruses for which the human immune system is too cumbersome or inefficient, by which it can be easily overwhelmed. Sometimes the immune system is provoked into an inflammatory reaction more damaging than the virus itself, as happens in the 'immunological' phase of Covid-19 pneumonia, when the very cells that are supposed to be attacking the virus begin to thicken and inflame the lungs.

When a virus has co-evolved among one population for thousands of years, there's a degree of familiarity and protection within that community. Smallpox, caused by the variola virus, was endemic in Europe and Asia right up to and through the early modern period, until vaccination became routine: babies would have taken in some antibodies with their mother's breast milk, and, although smallpox outbreaks were common, the population as a whole had been exposed to it frequently and so those epidemics were not as devastating for them as they were, for instance, for the indigenous populations in the Americas, who were exposed to the virus for the first time after the arrival of the European colonists. 'Herd immunity' would often be reached, when the proportion of the population who *had* been exposed was large enough to protect those who hadn't; the virus still spread, but more slowly than it otherwise would have done.

Similarly, there are degrees of immunity: if you suffered badly from chickenpox as a child, you would expect to be protected when exposed to it as an adult, but if you had it mildly you might have only a relatively muted antibody response, and remain vulnerable to a second attack. Nonetheless, that second attack will likely be less severe because of your previous exposure – your immune system will be more agile, better prepared, when it meets the virus next time around. By July 2020 it was being proposed that some people suffered only minimal illness with SARS-CoV-2 because of previous exposure to other coronaviruses. They're common pathogens, usually causing only mild cough and cold symptoms, so it would be surprising if there wasn't a degree of crossover immunity between different subtypes of the same virus.

The first known effective attempt to curtail the spread of a virus was made in China, where, in the tenth century, the scabs of someone who'd suffered only a mild case of smallpox began to be powdered and blown into the noses of children as young as five. The aim was to give the children a gentler version of the illness, provoking a reaction strong enough that it would confer immunity, but weak enough that recovery would be swift. Many children must have died when the procedure went wrong, but enough were saved that it seems to have been considered a gamble worth taking. By the seventeenth and eighteenth centuries, in the Ottoman Empire and sub-Saharan Africa, a similar procedure, later called 'variolation', had become widespread, in which the smallpox scab was not powdered but inserted under a nick in the skin. The recipient would go into quarantine (the word means 'forty days') during which, it was hoped, they would contract a mild case and develop subsequent immunity. The practice spread to England from 1718 thanks to Lady Mary Wortley Montagu, the writer, adventurer and wife of the British ambassador to Turkey, who had suffered from smallpox herself and had her son inoculated in the Ottoman fashion.

Like the Chinese method of blowing powdered scabs up the nose, variolation had grave risks. Nothing safer was devised until an English farmer called Benjamin Jesty, who had himself been variolated in the Ottoman way, noticed that two dairymaids of his acquaintance, Anne Notley and Mary Reade, appeared immune to the disease. Jesty made an elegant connection: that their immunity was related to their regular contact with a very similar disease to smallpox, cowpox. Using 'stocking needles' to scrape the udders of an infected cow he variolated his wife and two sons with these scabs (the word 'vaccination' comes from the Latin for cow, *vacca*). Jesty had had no medical training, he simply remembered the specifics of the procedure from his own variolation as a child.

Vaccination reached Scotland a few years later, after the English physician Edward Jenner – often credited with its invention – popularised Jesty's experiment and gave it international prestige. In a reverse of the pattern seen among the current anti-vax movement, it was more popular among the educated than the uneducated. At the close of the eighteenth century Sir John Sinclair observed in *The Statistical Account of Scotland* that 'Multitudes of the common people considered inoculation as criminal; – as an encroachment upon the prerogative of Providence'.

Smallpox remains the only virus humanity has managed to eradicate completely (though samples are retained, incomprehensibly, in disease control labs in both the US and Russia). It continued to rise and fall in epidemics across the globe throughout the nineteenth century and into the late twentieth century. The last case of major smallpox (*variola major*) to be recorded was in Bangladesh in 1975, and the last case of minor smallpox (*variola minor*) caught in the community was that of a Somalian hospital cook called Ali Maow Maalin, in 1977. Maalin subsequently became involved with the campaign to eradicate polio, and died in 2013 while carrying out a vaccination programme. 'Somalia was the last country with smallpox,' he said. 'I wanted to help ensure that we would not be the last place with polio, too.'

Maalin's wasn't, though, the last case of the disease – the story of *that* case is a cautionary reminder of the importance of absolute elimination of a dangerous virus through vaccination, and the precautions necessary if any viral material is to be stored long-term. Janet Parker was a medical photographer with an office at Birmingham Medical School adjacent to that of a virologist called Henry Bedson. It's still not known how she contracted smallpox from Bedson's laboratory, but in 1978, a few months after Maalin's recovery, she died of it. 'One infected person can easily spread the virus and start an epidemic anywhere,' wrote *The New York Times*, reporting on the story. 'The British [enquiry], headed by Prof. R. A. Shooter, concluded that Mrs Parker was infected either when the virus escaped through the air or was transferred to her by accidental contact with a visitor to the laboratory.'

Parker's mother Hilda, the last person in the world to catch smallpox from another human being, made a full recovery. Henry Bedson died a few days earlier than Parker, by suicide.

Edinburgh's Regional Infectious Diseases Unit (RIDU) is round the back of the city's Western General Hospital – a Victorian poorhouse turned infirmary which once stood among fields, but whose buildings have multiplied over the centuries in a kind of architectural mitosis, new structures, splitting, branching, metastasising over its once spacious grounds. The last time I'd been there was a while ago, after an unfortunate incident on nightshift. It was the witching hour, 4 a.m., when our core temperature is at its lowest and I'm always at my clumsiest. I'd just taken blood from a patient with Hepatitis C – a silent killer of a virus, then circulating at a high level among drug users in Edinburgh – and my trembling hands fumbled the dirty needle just as I withdrew it from the patient's vein. The needle snapped out of my fingers, flipped 180 degrees, and its contaminated point scratched the back of my ungloved hand. I cursed under my breath, suddenly wide awake, and ran from the patient's bedside to run the graze under a hot tap in the hope of bleeding out the virus before it took root in my body. I massaged the skin under the hot water for as long as my efforts could squeeze forth the slightest hint of blood. The incident was my own fault – the lack of gloves, the lack of care – and it was my own idiocy that I cursed. I'd only been doing the shift as a favour for someone else, and now I was condemned to months of blood tests and clinical reviews at the RIDU to see whether I'd contracted the virus. But in the end I was lucky, and was spared the harrowing and only partially successful treatments then available for Hepatitis C.

This time round, though, I was there to meet some of the team involved in Edinburgh's trials of a new SARS-CoV-2 vaccine, which was being tested on volunteer healthcare workers. I was curious to know how such an immense vaccine study, with global implications and the very highest of stakes, had managed to get off the ground in a matter of weeks, and all against the background of coping with the spring start of the pandemic. The early development of the vaccine had been in Oxford, where coronavirus proteins had been inserted into a virus that causes cough and cold symptoms in chimpanzees. In an echo of Benjamin Jesty using a cow virus to cure a human one, the aim was to neutralise a bat virus afflicting humans, using one that prefers chimps: turning our vulnerability to zoonotic infections into a possible solution to them. As I read over the patient information leaflet for the vaccine study I saw how that principle established by the Chinese – of using old, dried smallpox scabs from mild cases to produce a weaker infection – had been developed for the new coronavirus vaccine. It had been genetically altered, the leaflet reassured me, so that it couldn't grow in humans. Genes coding for the sugared protein spike on the surface of the SARS-CoV-2 virus had been inserted. 'We are hoping to make the body recognise and develop an immune response to the Spike protein,' the leaflet said, 'that will help stop the

SARS-CoV-2 virus from entering human cells and therefore prevent infection.'

From the outside, RIDU appears as a double layer of prefabs, grey and yellow, with all the charm and architectural interest of a breeze block. Inside it carries the imprimatur of the era in which it was conceived: mahogany veneer doors, fittings and furnishings in a matching brown plastic, faded signage. But, as with so much of the British National Health Service, the age and décor of the buildings belie the sophistication of the work that goes on inside, and the affection of the staff for those same buildings.

Becky Sutherland, with whom I had been in touch in June over the school closures letter, is one of the consultants in RIDU, now coordinating the Edinburgh cohort of the Oxford Coronavirus vaccine trial. I knew that Becky had hardly had a day off since February: initially managing all the swab positive Covid-19 patients in hospital while at the same time helping track down and isolate the contacts of every case. Then came 13 March, and the regrettable about-turn in national efforts to contain the virus – overnight, it was announced that there would no more hospital admissions of positive cases, no contact tracing, and swabbing would be confined to those deemed unwell enough to need admission to hospital. This was the period of promoting the idea of natural 'herd immunity', aiming to slow transmission but allowing it to move through the population without overwhelming the NHS. That abrupt shift in policy was, in retrospect, a mistake, and Becky's frustration was palpable when I brought it up: governments across the UK spent months playing catch-up. If contact tracing had been implemented from the start it might have been possible to avert the first lengthy nationwide lockdown. Even at this late stage of the first wave, without a vaccine, isolating every case was the only way society was ever going to get back to something approaching normal.

Becky showed the way down the corridor to her office, a
sagging give to the floorboards putting a spring in our steps.
Inside, there was a chair where I could sit at a two-metre distance from her desk, and it was a relief to dispense with the
mask. Above the desk were crayon drawings by her children,
charts and spreadsheets, and a postcard of a medieval plague
doctor wearing a hood stuffed with medicinal herbs (which
reminded me that I'd recently heard of people dripping lav-
ender and tea tree oil into their masks). I asked her how she
got involved.

'I worked in Oxford once with some of the organisers, and
they rang me up. It seemed like such an important study that
I said yes, of course.' For the vaccine programme to work,
two things were going to be needed: firstly, a population
that was willing to volunteer and actively engage with being
monitored week in week out for as much as a year; and sec-
ondly, that population had to be more than usually exposed
to coronavirus. Healthcare staff ticked both boxes. Exhaus-
tive tests would be required, with participants giving blood
samples to check their genetic profiles, their immune respon-
siveness, their antibody levels. Becky urgently needed to find
twenty doctors and thirty nurses who would determine each
volunteer's suitability, exclude those with contraindications,
give the vaccines by injection, review the volunteers and
swab them, take blood tests, and also be available to take
part in a 24-hour on-call rota. This was crucial so that if any
trial participant felt unwell – either with symptoms of Covid-
19, or with some kind of reaction to the vaccine itself – they
would swiftly be able to access someone on the team who
could see them urgently.

'It's amazing how much my colleagues have given to the
project,' she said. 'With so much clinical work shut down in
anticipation of the first wave, there were plenty of clinicians
who weren't busy. But many of the doctors and nurses who

came forward to help us on their days off come from the busiest specialties: they're in A&E, acute medicine; our own registrars in infectious disease were great, the orthopaedic staff, too. You realise there are people working in the NHS who are just deeply selfless, they want to help in any way they can. And if that means they give up their days off to join the effort, they just do it.'

Becky introduced me to Sheila Morris, a nurse who coordinates and supervises clinical research and someone who has spent almost forty years investigating how we can manage infectious disease better. She began her career during the 1980s HIV/AIDS epidemic. 'Sheila was there at the beginning,' said Becky, 'up in the City Hospital, when GPs like Roy Robertson were roaming the streets like cowboys, saving the drug users of Edinburgh.' Roy Robertson was a GP in Muirhouse, one of the most deprived wards of the city, who played an important part, first in recognising, and then in responding to, the HIV epidemic in Edinburgh. In the mid-1990s he'd been among my tutors on an inspirational GP attachment that influenced my own decision to become a GP. A collage of photographs hung by Sheila's office door, glossy pictures of her and her colleagues, laughing through the calamity. Papers were piled high on her desk. 'My career has taken me through two pandemics,' she told me, 'HIV and now coronavirus. I don't plan on seeing a third.'

Sheila said the research intensity of the past few months had been like nothing she had ever seen, even at the height of the HIV crisis in the 1980s. The number of trials coming out now was dizzying: the RECOVERY Trial for those needing critical care support; the PHOSP-COVID trial, looking into post-hospitalisation and the long-term effects of having suffered from Covid-19; the PRINCIPLE trial for anyone over 65 with symptoms early in their illness; and now the Oxford vaccine trial. It was clear more would be coming down the line through the coming months. There had been numerous twists and challenges in the course of setting up the Oxford trial – the protocol had been changed seven times since it was first sent out, and the study organisers had had to be flexible. I was reminded of Rankin Barr's perspective on how quickly the housing crisis in the city had been solved when vested interests were put aside, and bureaucratic barriers dropped. So much was possible when professionals like him, like Sheila and Becky, were given permission to be pragmatic.

It was far from certain that the Oxford vaccine would provoke a strong or durable immune reaction that could protect the population. But the social, medical and economic situation brought about by the pandemic was desperate. As I left RIDU I felt buoyed, inspired, thinking about how dedicated groups of clinicians and scientists all over the world were collaborating to find any kind of solution that might help us get back to normality.

Coronavirus vaccines have proven particularly difficult to produce for a number of reasons. Firstly, the viruses mutate quickly, meaning that by the time the vaccine is developed, trialled, cleared for use and distributed, the virus itself may well have moved on, and the vaccine that has been so painstakingly produced will no longer offer protection. Then there's the fact that, as far as the body is concerned, the theatre of action for coronaviruses is *outside*, in the passages of the nose, throat and lungs where it's more difficult for antibodies to reach. Thirdly, when we do manage to generate immunity against common cold viruses it's often only temporary, lasting months rather than years, and so, although there's a hope that having people vaccinated against coronavirus will make repeat infections much milder in terms of their effects, that's by no means certain.

A fourth more worrying problem was shown in the efforts twenty years ago to develop a coronavirus vaccine against SARS-CoV-1. Ferrets given a vaccine against that coronavirus developed immunity rapidly, but when they subsequently became infected by SARS-CoV-1, their own immune system seemed to react not just by attacking the virus but by attacking their own livers. Mice immunised against SARS-CoV-1 developed a kind of allergic response that was as damaging as the infection itself. This is the paradox, and the fear, at the heart of the way Covid-19 afflicts the body: that on its own the virus can inflame and damage the lungs and other organs, but at the same time the body's very response to that virus can on occasion prove even more dangerous.

One of the fascinating outcomes of the Oxford vaccine trial so far has been how many participants seem to carry a level of protection to the virus, though they have no detectable circulating antibodies. Only 6 per cent of Becky's cohort seemed to have developed a 'humoral' response to the virus (the terminology used to describe antibodies in the blood, recalling the 'humours' of Greek medicine), even though many had worked on Covid wards through the peak of the pandemic. Their bodies seemed instead to have mounted a purely 'cellular' response through T-cells, a type of white blood cell that doesn't make antibodies, as opposed to B-cells, which do. There are four types of T-cells: they can be 'helpers' of B-cells; 'killers' of infected body cells; they can drive inflammation in the tissues of the body; or they can modulate the immune response to prevent the kind of immune storm that becomes self-defeating. 'But it's still too early to say,' Becky had told me. 'We're starting to see some participants swab positive, and it'll be fascinating to see whether they turn out to be more protected than the others.'

But as coronavirus transmission in Scotland continued to fall, the study was going to come up against a welcome problem – there wasn't enough Covid-19 around to see whether those who had been vaccinated were more protected than others. In Oxford a call had gone out for young, healthy volunteers who'd been vaccinated to *expose* themselves to the virus. Becky told me that there were branches of this study being set up in Brazil, the USA and Kenya.

Talk in the clinic with colleagues and patients was often about how long it would be until we have a vaccine – and I realised just how much vaccines have transformed the practice of medicine, and all of our lives. But at the same time, studies were being published showing that fewer than 70 per cent of British people would accept a vaccination against SARS-CoV-2 – less than the level required to produce herd immunity, which for many other viruses is between 80 and 95 per cent. In the course of my medical career I'd seen the dismal effects of a drop in vaccination rates, particularly of Measles Mumps and Rubella (MMR): diseases had resurged that, throughout my earlier medical training, I'd assumed had been consigned to the history books. I still meet parents today anxious about MMR and autism, though the connection has been utterly disproven. As similarly groundless conspiracy theories about Covid vaccination began to circulate on the internet I realised how much the near-universal vaccination of the late twentieth century has bred a kind of complacency, at least in the West.

It had been a year or two since I'd last seen Simon; he was a young man in his mid-twenties, a software designer who wore old-style NHS specs, a perpetual three-day stubble and his hair tied back in a short ponytail. He had a variety of skin conditions: eczema, psoriasis and acne, and all of our conversations had been about one of those three, about finding a balance of therapy whereby the treatment for one wouldn't upset the others. So it was a surprise when he rang me up to say he wanted to talk about vaccination. 'How so?' I asked him.

'My parents didn't believe in immunisations,' he said, 'so I haven't had any. With all this Covid around, I'm starting to think that maybe that wasn't such a good idea.'

Simon was a child when the now discredited MMR conspiracy was in circulation, but his parents had made their decision before the story broke. He'd been lucky; because the majority of his classmates and community had been vaccinated he hadn't suffered unduly. I thought of some of the other unvaccinated children I knew of who hadn't been so fortunate: one in twenty children with measles develop pneumonia, although only about one in a thousand develop the most serious complication, encephalitis (a viral infection of brain cells). About two children in a thousand will die of measles. I arranged for Simon to come in and discuss it more face to face, and get started on his own belated vaccination schedule.

There are all sorts of reasons that people refuse vaccination, either for themselves or for their children. In her book *Calling the Shots*, the American sociologist Jennifer Reich, who has studied vaccine refusal, cited an odd paradox: that among her US study group, parents who chose to delay having children had higher levels of education than those who had children early, but that they were more likely to reject vaccination. Reich concluded that their refusal was predicated on considering themselves 'experts on their own children' who didn't wish to take advice from other (medical) experts.

According to Reich, members of the communities she studied had a lower sense of their responsibility to one another than in previous decades, while at the same time low levels of childhood illness through earlier decades had promoted an overconfidence in the power of children to fight off infectious disease. Awareness of environmental toxins, and distrust of pharmaceutical companies, was common. She also noted that 'healthism' had become widespread among certain elite and professional groups. It was a new word to me, describing the belief that healthy eating and exercise are enough to protect against infectious diseases.

Reich doesn't have any time for parent-blaming, and points out that it's generally counterproductive to portray vaccine-refusing parents as 'foolish or ignorant at best, and sometimes even delusional or selfish'. In her book's introduction she says simply that she had all her own children vaccinated, because 'I trust that vaccines are mostly safe and I accept that we can each absorb minimal risk to protect those in our community who are most vulnerable'.

With Simon I went through the vaccines he'd missed out on, and began to discuss which ones he should start with, booking in his follow-up appointments with Geraldine, one of our two superb practice nurses. The latest iteration of the UK immunisation schedule covers some twenty-one different pathogens, from the diphtheria, tetanus and polio that we begin with at just eight weeks of age – devastating illnesses that once made infancy the most perilous phase of life – through to the last one currently on the schedule at age 70, when the vaccine against shingles, a painful, blistering recurrence of the chickenpox virus, is given. The schedule of immunisations offers a spectrum of protection, and a degree of freedom from avoidable suffering that was unthinkable to previous generations, built on the unseen work of thousands of doctors, nurses, scientists and volunteers.

*

As the 'new normal' became more established, I began to see the late effects of the long periods of isolation that so many of my patients had endured. Mr Malcolm lives just a few doors down from the surgery. I remember an encounter with him just as lockdown came in: he'd turned up at the surgery door without an appointment, in a fog of dementia confusion and unable to say why he was there or what was bothering him. I sat him down, got him a glass of water and went to phone the number of the person we had recorded as his next of kin – who happened to be a granddaughter. I could hear children's cries in the background of the call, excited and cheerful ones, as well as anguished and outraged ones. But the granddaughter, Kirsty, was calm – her voice held concern for her granddad, honestly conveyed, and she didn't sound harassed or keen to get off the phone to attend to her own children.

Mr Malcolm had been wandering more and more, she said, and she was worried how he'd cope with the lockdown when she, along with everyone else in the country, had been asked to stay away from the elderly and isolate in their own homes. 'You've got to understand something about my granddad,' Kirsty said. 'He *lives* for his great-grandchildren. You should see his face when he sees them – and theirs when they see him – they just light up.'

At the time I hoped the lockdown wouldn't go on too long, that Mr Malcolm would find ways of seeing those great-grandchildren despite it. But his home was a small apartment with no garden even to wave at them from. The national messaging at the time was of the vital importance that everyone comply with the advice – coronavirus was spreading fast with an R_0 number of 2–3, and unless everyone complied, dementia or not, the consequences would be dire.

Most of us carry a hidden antechamber of anything we're preparing to say, some preparatory room of the linguistic mind in which we try out phrases and gauge their potential effect, and in that mental space I felt a phrase begin to form: something about priorities and the end of life; how Mr M – surely now in his last few years and with so little left of the richness and complexity that give most of our lives sense and purpose – might well feel that the permission to go on seeing his great-grandchildren would trump any risk of contracting, and dying, from coronavirus. But as the phrasing assembled itself, I realised that to even suggest it might constitute an unfair burden on Kirsty. Mr Malcolm no longer had the capacity to make that kind of decision for himself – his dementia was too far advanced – and so I'd be leaving the decision to Kirsty and the rest of the family. If he went on to die of the virus as a consequence of dandling those great-grandchildren on his knee, the whole family might come to feel an intolerable burden of guilt.

I didn't hear much from Mr Malcolm or from Kirsty until early July, when elements of lockdown were easing for some, and there were murmurings of shielded patients being able to mix again with their families. By then Mr Malcolm had been at home alone for nearly four months.

A call from Kirsty was the alert. He had been listless and anxious on the telephone, agitated, and she asked me tentatively if I'd call on him. 'I'll go round and see him,' I said, 'and get back to you later this morning.'

How we pass our days is, in the end, how we pass our lives, and the manner in which we surround ourselves with things reveals what we most value. I've picked my way through squalid slums in which books of astonishing erudition and intellectual range are stacked from floor to ceiling, and between those stacks of books narrow passageways linking armchair, kitchen, bedroom and bathroom, like the desire lines that animals press down into long grass. I've visited lonesome homes whose rooms are like sterile shopfronts or show houses, where it feels as if the only love left is the one of keeping up with the neighbours. I like the messy, homely places best, with shoes kicked off in the doorways and the walls a patchy collage of lists, tickets, scrawled drawings and pictures chosen for their memories, not their quality.

Mr Malcolm's home was a manifestation of the kind of love that only a few are lucky enough to enjoy. Every wall and every surface was a gallery of family photos; from the looks of the hairstyles and clothes and the manner in which they were taken, the images extended across six or seven decades. There are different kinds of wealth, after all. And though those clothing styles changed, and the fashions of professional photographers and their studios evolved, in the toothy smiles and the folds at the corner of the eyes I could discern the same family, running through four generations. It was a pleasure to note in one image from the 1970s a man and a woman hugging each other, in flowered shirts and hippy hair, and then to see those same faces evolve through the eighties, nineties, changing into suits and summer dresses, gain and lose perms, gather children around them, then watch the once-long hair turn thin and grey. To see in other photographs those same children grown into young men and women at their own weddings, graduations, birth-day parties.

As I followed him into his sitting room, Mr Malcolm walked through this gallery of family memory and seemed less a patriarch than the drifting spirit of the already-departed; the only thing that would tether him back to life would be if I pointed out a particular photograph, and the image would forge a connection the way a steeple calls down a blade of lightning. A smile would break out. 'That's my grandson,' he'd say. 'William – he does something with computers.' Or 'That's me! Believe it or not, that's me not long after I was first married.'

I called Kirsty, explained how I'd found her grandad, and began to pick my way through a difficult conversation about compromise: his need of his family and its sustaining power, and their fear of infecting him. 'You've done so well,' I said, 'you've really kept him safe. But I think we're getting to the point when we have to ask what we're keeping him safe *for.*' I was relieved to hear that they'd restarted their visits.

A welcome consequence of the pandemic has been an easing of communication between hospital consultants and doctors like me in the community. With their own outpatient clinics cancelled, many specialists were instantly accessible on the phone, or by email, to give advice. An Edinburgh oncologist, Lesley Dawson, had asked if I'd give a talk to the 'Grand Round' of NHS Lothian, usually held at Western General Hospital and attended over a lunchtime by hospital specialists, but which would now have to be delivered online – the same forum at which I'd heard Andrew Watson describe the surge in new adult psychosis brought on by the lockdown. The new format meant that, for the first time, hospital clinicians, GPs and district nurses could attend the same meetings. The fall in cases and in deaths gave a kind of respite or breathing space, and I was happy to give the talk. I'm no spokeperson for the politics of general practice – only for my own practice – and so I asked Carey Lunan, president of the Royal College of General Practitioners Scotland and a clinician working in one of Edinburgh's most deprived communities, if she'd join me to offer a second, more diplomatic political perspective, and was relieved when she agreed.

The talk we gave was called 'General Practice & Covid-19: A Personal and Political Perspective'. In Orkney I'd spent some hours figuring out what I would say, and asked a few friends who are hospital consultants what they'd most like to hear about. Many of them said they still had little idea of how GPs had responded to the pandemic, and what changes had been imposed on the ways that we work. 'We don't know what it's reasonable to expect you to do,' Lesley had said. A friend who is a renal physician put it more bluntly: 'Just tell us what you do all day.'

I'm no fan of giving online talks: I don't like the delays, the glitches, the inability to read the room – being unable to hear the coughs and restlessness that indicate when a change in tone is needed, or the converse, the murmurs and nods that tell you you're on the right track. I don't like the way there's no way of acknowledging, in your delivery, that there are 500 people in the audience as opposed to five. There were 300 'in' the audience for Carey's and my talk, though there might as well have been three for all the atmosphere it had, delivered from my own front room. I went through the changes we'd been obliged to adopt in general practice through the pandemic: the switch to remote consulting; telephone triage; the terror of March as the cases were climbing; the relief of May as they began to fall – even as cases and deaths worldwide continued to soar. I explained the pattern of the working day back in January, and how much of our work was divided between mental health, managing long-term conditions, assessing kids with fevers and rashes, delivering end of life care, and that crucial 'gatekeeper' role of the British GP: assessing any worrying symptoms that might represent cancer or another serious illness, and getting them promptly investigated. I outlined a typical day with all its calls, correspondence and visits, and touched on the transformation of healthcare for the homeless people of the city, as well as how well I'd seen rural communities in Orkney respond to and protect themselves against the virus.

In general practice we faced the same problems as hospitals with regard to clinics opening up again: how to limit the numbers in our waiting rooms; and though supplies of PPE were much healthier, they weren't sufficient to allow us to return to normal. Admitting the miseries of the past few months was something I was glad to be able to emphasise, asking colleagues to acknowledge how awful much of it had been, and flashing up the wellbeing checklists that were going up in hospital corridors and changing rooms across the country. 'Acknowledge one thing that was difficult about today and let it go,' said one. 'Consider three things that went well.'

But the final slide was less solemn, though no less true, sent to me by a colleague during the peak in April. It was a photograph of the kind of DIY sign an Evangelical church might put up, but repurposed to spell out a different message, not quite as uplifting: 'Whoever said one person can't change the world never ate an undercooked bat.'

In mid-July the US passed 3.5 million cases, and 150,000 deaths, while globally the virus continued to spread. There were steepening graphs of cumulative cases from the USA, Brazil, Chile, India and South Africa, and though the death rate was flattening off in the USA, in Brazil it showed no sign of slowing. In the UK, from a peak of around 6,000 new infections every day we were down to just 445. The figures were improving so much I hoped it wouldn't lead to complacency.

On my bike ride into work, the cygnets I had passed each morning on the canal since May were down to just five now, getting bigger and more ungainly, unable to clamber on to the backs of their parents. My approach didn't bring as much panic as before – they paddled serenely to the far side of the water. After four months of being barred to the public, the middle of July saw the front door of my practice being unlocked. It felt as if the occasion demanded a ceremony, but in the end I just took down the 'No Entry' signs and clicked off the snib lock. Janis, the practice manager, prepared a new series of signs. Patients would no longer be obliged to address their queries to the front window, though they would still be asked to stick to a series of yellow footprint signs, spaced two metres apart. I brought in a drill from home and bolted sanitiser dispensers on to the corridor walls, and a perspex screen to the front of the reception desk.

With the front door unlocked, it was as if a literal and metaphorical draft of fresh air had begun to blow back into the clinic. It was not quite enough to make us feel that we could breathe easily, but it gave us hope that, despite the local outbreaks, the ongoing quarantine for holidaymakers, the dire predictions for the winter ahead, the unresolved question of how the coming flu season would interact with coronavirus, the job itself had not changed beyond recognition, and we could still attempt to practise the kind of medicine we were trained to do.

The people I brought in to consult with face to face, rather than down a videolink or telephone wire, were beginning to resolve into three principal categories. The first were those whose problem might flag an early sign of cancer, or something similarly devastating: the breast lumps; the bleeding from the bowel; the dry cough that just wouldn't settle; the slipped disc in the back, pushing on the spine and threatening permanent paralysis or incontinence. The second category were joint injections – through April, May and June, I'd been dosing all those with worn-out knees or inflamed shoulders with escalating quantities of painkillers. This felt wrong, given that more and more drugs lead inevitably to more and more side effects, but the obligation to keep people safe and at home trumped that concern. Now, slowly, I began to see those patients again in the clinic, pass a needle into that troublesome shoulder or knee to dampen the agony with a vial of steroids. And though the pandemic had illustrated just how much a crisis in healthcare relegates mental illness to second place, the third category of patients I began to see in person again were those with complex mental health issues; those for whom months of phone calls and tweaking of sedatives, antipsychotics and antidepressants had proven insufficient to soothe their minds. By mid-July, it was becoming increasingly clear that what was needed was not more medicines, websites or helplines, but human contact – sharing space, not just disembodied words and ideas.

From the science of Covidology it was emerging that what kills people in that awful second phase of infection, just as the majority are beginning their recovery, is as much a disease of the blood vessels as a disease of the lungs. The virus enters body cells through binding to the ACE-2 protein, involved in the maintenance of blood pressure – one of the mechanisms that helps finely calibrate the blood flow through our intricate, miraculous net of capillaries that nourish and sustain the body, gauging each tissue's requirement for oxygen and apportioning blood accordingly. Through that frightening first peak in March and April, our attention was focussed on the virus's effect on the lungs with good reason, because it was the failure of the lungs to adequately convey oxygen into the blood that was so often proving to be deadly. But there was increasing evidence that this occurred not solely through the virus's effect on lung tissue but on blood flow in the lungs, an effect also seen elsewhere in the body. Some balance or harmony of body circulation was being disturbed, with fatal consequences.

Changes to blood flow are of course most visible in the

skin, and back in March the first report on those changes had surfaced from the small town of Lecco, in Lombardy, where a group of dermatologists had been drafted in to the front line of providing medical care through the crisis engulfing northern Italy. One of them, Sebastiano Recalcati, noticed the frequency with which his Covid-19 patients developed odd skin rashes. His report has no photographs – unusual in a journal of dermatology. 'We visited directly or indirectly (because of the high risk of contagion and the lack of protective masks),' Recalcati explained. 'No clinical images were performed because of the high risk to infect other patients, introducing a photographic device in a restricted room ...' One in five patients had rashes of one kind or another, but the severity of the rash was no indication of the severity of the disease. The tone and language of medical journals is for the most part aggressively bland and distant, all emotion stripped from their syntax, but in Recalcati's report you can sense the oppressive, fearful atmosphere then suffocating the hospitals of Italy.

A month later, on 29 April, a group of Spanish dermatologists collated a countrywide study and published it in the *British Journal of Dermatology*, describing 375 patients with skin changes, all seen through the first peak of the epidemic in Spain. The variety of ways the virus had affected the skin was startling: chilblains, nettle rash and blistering were common, but also seen was the kind of rashes ordinarily associated with meningitis, with dark blooms of clotted blood vessels mottling the surface. In some cases – around one in twenty of their sample – patches of skin had simply died away as the blood supply to them had choked off. The patients afflicted by this 'necrosis' had the highest fatality rate among all the patients assessed by the study – only around one in five of them survived.

In my own clinic I'd seen examples of this strange effect

on the blood vessels of the skin. The toes, being furthest from the heart and subject to the weight of gravity pulling blood towards the feet, are often where disturbances in blood flow become manifest. Some of my patients developed chilblains alongside their Covid cough and fever, as if they'd been marching through the snow with wet, chilled feet rather than living through the warmest, driest April on record. And, as Recalcati had noticed, the severity of these rashes seemed to have no bearing on the severity of the disease – none of the people I saw affected by 'Covid toes' needed to go to hospital, and all were relatively mildly affected by the virus: a few days of fever, a week or two of cough, some fatigue, then they bounced back to normal. The skin changes, though, stayed – by July it was still possible to make out the faintest of stigmata over the skin of the toes, a shadow left by the passage of the virus.

There were other long-term repercussions and, through July, as restrictions eased little by little and my clinic began to open up, I began seeing more and more of them. The young woman whose only symptom of Covid-19 had been a sudden loss of smell. Twelve weeks on she felt well, but her sense of smell and of taste had not returned. The 25-year-old footballer who, four months on, was still suffering episodic pains in the chest. The fifty-something runner who, eight weeks on, was still breathless walking up the hill to my clinic, and struggled to complete a four-kilometre circuit on level ground. The 60-year-old woman who'd had cough and fever badly at the time, and again, had never needed assessment in hospital. One day she called me: she'd bought an oxygen sensor online and wanted to know the normal range. 'Well for you, I'd think 96 per cent or so,' I told her. 'Oh,' she replied, 'because I can't get a reading higher than 93 per cent.' Whatever process the virus had triggered in her lungs had yet to run its course, though she'd long since stopped being infectious and in other ways had returned to normal.

These 'long Covid' symptoms were so widespread that, in my area, a dedicated phone number was set up to offer advice, the service staffed by physiotherapists practised in lung recovery who were able to explain to frightened patients what was emerging as normal with this disease, what the trajectory of convalescence might look like, and when to be concerned and seek help. I phoned the number myself on behalf of one of my patients, left a message with a telephonist, who arranged for the physiotherapist to call me back. 'We've had many callers who've experienced ongoing chest "tightness" and generally more effort to inhale,' the physio, Claudia, said when she got back to me. 'Unusually for a physiotherapist, I'm generally discouraging people from vigorous exercise and encouraging more rest and less activity whilst they are still symptomatic.' She sent me a booklet to hand out to affected patients, which explained in language that was both clear and concise how to improve their exercise tolerance, how to manage episodes of breathlessness, how to clear their chests of phlegm. It began with a list of just a few 'long Covid' effects, recognisable as a collection of symptoms seen in other kinds of post-viral fatigue:

- Muscle weakness and joint stiffness
- Extreme tiredness (fatigue) and a lack of energy
- Loss of appetite and weight loss
- Sleep problems
- Problems with mental abilities – for example, not being able to remember some events and think clearly, and being forgetful
- Changes in your mood, or anxiety or depression
- Nightmares or flashbacks
- Breathlessness
- Cough

For many, it was the fatigue that was most debilitating, as if the body's response to the stress of beating coronavirus was to retreat into some kind of physiological safe mode in which exhaustion was pervasive, work was impossible, and the only option was to rest.

In conversation with patients I'm often struck by society's ubiquitous work ethic, an ethic which tends towards an impatience with convalescence which can itself be harmful. If you feel in need of rest then it's usually because your body requires it. But with each day of bed rest we lose a little strength and confidence; withdrawal from the world can harm our sense of mental equilibrium and of our rootedness in community. For every day immobile in bed, ITU patients lose 2 per cent of their muscle mass; those recovering from coronavirus risk the same kind of 'deconditioning' from inactivity. And offering advice to people with this kind of post-viral fatigue is often a difficult balancing act because of the inherent paradox that for each patient will require a subtly different resolution. To keep the body moving it's usually necessary to keep revisiting the edge of what's possible in terms of effort, in order to maintain strength and confidence. But push too hard and that effort can miscarry into a deeper and more enduring exhaustion – what the physiotherapists of rehabilitation called a cycle of 'boom and bust'.

The difficulties of lockdown had shown just how much we are social beings; for long Covid sufferers entering months of slow and often challenging recovery, it was painful to see the communities around them return to something approaching normality, albeit masked and distanced, while they continued to endure an isolation and quarantine imposed not by the government but by the illness.

*

Earlier in July quarantine rules had been relaxed for people arriving in the UK from seventy-five different countries: the US was not included, but Spain, France, Germany and other European countries were. The re-opening of society was inherently risky, but just as socially necessary: government figures showed that over 600,000 people had lost their jobs since the pandemic began, many of them in the tourist and airline industries. The rates of infection in Spain were rising again, while in South Africa alarm was being raised over the huge discrepancy between the official death toll from Covid-19 and the number of excess deaths for the time of year. The WHO marked six months since they'd first raised the alarm over the evolving pandemic by warning that its duration would be 'lengthy'. I was increasingly anxious that for these few weeks of summer freedom we'd receive in exchange long months of winter lockdown, but the alternative – of banning foreign travel or policing quarantine effectively, as in China – seemed politically impossible.

Among my practice population in Edinburgh of close to 4,000 people, three had died of Covid-19, three or four times that had been hospitalised, and scores had made a full recovery – about the same proportions as had been affected UK-wide. On the last day of July I listened to a newsreader announce the 'excess death' figures for Europe – the number of deaths over and above normal for the time of year, a statistic thought to be more reliable than recorded Covid-19 deaths, in that it counts the deaths of people who hadn't been tested, as well as the impact the pandemic had had in contributing to the deaths of people who were unable or unwilling to access usual medical care. Across Europe, England was worst, Spain second, Scotland third. Italy's figures weren't available. There were angry exchanges on the radio;

politicians pleading for understanding and stressing the incomparability of different countries' figures.

I saw a terrific play once, *Cockpit* by Bridget Boland, written in 1947, which explores our common humanity in the face of infectious disease. The Edinburgh theatre I saw it in was transformed into a historically rendered provincial German playhouse, repurposed as a camp for refugees and displaced persons and run by British soldiers. The soldiers were attempting to organise the different refugees into groups who'd be able to travel home together. But some groups kept refusing to be associated with others, and the dialogue brought up ancient enmities and blood feuds. No one would agree with the British plans for repatriation until one refugee died of what appeared to be bubonic plague.

The soldiers locked down the theatre – no one was allowed in or out, including the guards (and members of the audience). With the common threat of the plague bacillus to fight against, the residents' common humanity asserted itself, and the anger and historic hatreds melted away. Jew or Pole, Russian or English, they were all equally susceptible to the infection, and would be obliged to face the outbreak together. There developed a shared purpose in the face of the disease that I recognised in the cross-party unity of those months of lockdown, the acceptance of government restrictions by almost everyone in society, the NHS rainbows, the clapping for key workers, the community art, lines of painted pebbles, and repeated affirmations that together we would get through this. *Cockpit* sees an opera singer among the refugees sing an aria, further dissolving any divisions; that accord, provoked by disease, was heightened somehow by song, poetry, by reverence for the beauty and the power of art. It was cautionary and at the same time inspirational to see how easily prejudice could be swept aside. And this virus, too, has revealed our common humanity, our interdependence, our shared frailties and the power that we might wield if we choose to collaborate rather than compete.

Towards the end of the play, the diagnosis of 'plague' turned out to be a wrong one, and the threat that had united everyone in the theatre was revealed as illusory. Immediately the ethnic furies and ancient grudges erupted again, just as, now that the peak of infections had passed, politicians were back to shouting over one another again, throwing around accusations of blame.

That same day, 31 July, I heard the details of another change to the protocol of the vaccine study, the eighth: all recipients were to receive a booster dose. One dose of the vaccine seemed to confer some kind of protection against the virus, but not enough, apparently, to prevent reinfection. There were rumours that, following the success of the lockdown, case numbers were on the rise again across Europe, and on 27 July the government had reimposed a fourteen-day quarantine on travellers returning from Spain. In the weeks to come, France, Belgium and the Netherlands would join the list.

PART III

REPRISE

REINFECTION

*'[T]he disease was ... only frozen up, it would like a frozen river
have returned to its usual force and current when it thawed ...'*
Daniel Defoe
A Journal of the Plague Year

The reprise of a piece of music is rarely the same notation
repeated exactly; it's often fleshed out, deepened in repeti-
tion, elaborated with harmonies. Even when the bars are
repeated, the listener, having heard those themes before,
anticipates and responds differently to melodies heard a second time. We'd been through a crescendo in the early months
of the year, when the intensity of transmission forced an
almost deafening transformation of the way that medicine
was practised in the community, then a diminuendo through
the early months of the summer, as space began to open up
in our lives, and we could begin to take stock of all that had
changed.

In August, as holidaymakers began to return and cases of
the virus began to climb again, it was as if society itself was
undergoing a slow reinfection – a relapse. The themes of my
working days were like a musical piece I'd heard before, inti-
mately familiar, but altered by experience, by the ability to
anticipate what was coming. In August the virus had – with
the exceptions of some local pockets of infection – retreated
and, while we knew that it was still there, that the autumn

and winter might bring it sweeping back with more deaths, more lockdown, there was also the hope that this time it might be different. We thought we knew the tune this time.

That anticipation was echoed across society: in hospital medicine, in supermarket logistics, in government planning, in business resilience. One of the themes of those August days was that I dared to feel more hopeful of society's ability to cope with the growing second wave of infections. I've tried in these pages to show some ways in which our communities have always been shaped by infectious disease, but it had been so long – over a century – since a comparable viral pandemic had struck, that a complacency had begun to build both within my profession and within the government departments tasked with pandemic preparation. It was a complacency that we had been rudely shaken out of, and my optimism carried the knowledge of all the hard work that had been done to make up for the time that had been lost. We had available testing for anyone with symptoms, we had procedures and technology to manage the majority of patients at a distance, and – crucially – we now had enough PPE.

On 1 August the last of the shielding advice had been rescinded, though a few of my own patients were unconvinced and chose to stay home. Pedalling to and from the clinic I saw that the cygnets by the canal were fully grown – though still brown in their plumage, white feathers were beginning to show as they ruffled their wings. At the weekend and evening service it had become much easier to manage the potential coronavirus cases – to arrange prompt testing, to explain the rules for self-isolation and quarantine, to arrange face to face assessments in a dedicated clinic.

One Saturday night I was out in the car, travelling around the north side of the city to visit anyone who needed to see a GP but couldn't leave their home. An old man who'd been coughing up blood met me at his door, leaning on his zimmer frame. 'I'm Tommy Black,' he said, as I stood on his garden path, tying on my mask, 'or what's left o' 'im.' A 45-year-old woman in a Georgian palace of a home, rolling around in bed with the agony of impacted gallstones. A 60-year-old man with an acute paranoid psychosis – he'd been separated from his wife for many years, and she'd called us because his text messages to her, which had become increasingly bizarre in the months since the first lockdown, had that day mentioned alien interference, transmitters in his electric sockets and CIA surveillance of his home. I arrived to find him crouched in a corner of his bedroom, duvet pulled up to his chin. It took an hour of patient persuasion before I got him to agree to go up to the psychiatric hospital.

Throughout August in any normal year, the population of Edinburgh doubles as the city's summer festivals ignite one by one like firecrackers: the Fringe, the International Festival, the Book Festival, the Mela, the Art Festival. But on a Saturday night in August 2020, the city seemed to have been replaced by a dystopia: there was a stark emptiness to the streets; the pavements were desolate; many bars and restaurants were still closed. Bus shelters and billboards recalled happier festival years, as if trying to remind everyone that there is another world waiting for us on the other side of the pandemic – a sweeter world, charged with the knowledge of what could be lost. Outside the few nightclubs and bars that were open I saw bouncers in patterned and sloganeering masks – worn as a nod to individuality, or as a sly rebellion. Any masks were welcome: they spoke of a reassuring conformity to the rules and acknowledged the seriousness of the threat we still faced.

The months of the first national lockdown, of struggling

against the virus and the measures taken against it, had been difficult for everyone in the caring professions. Hundreds had lost their lives. But they made me appreciate with greater intensity the importance of the human connections that we make in our communities, in our families, between colleagues, between doctor and patient. As I'd become accustomed to seeing the faces of my patients only from behind a mask, and they'd in turn regarded me from behind their own masks, I yearned for the beauty and straightforward facility with which medicine was practised before the pandemic broke.

Time is never circular, though occasionally it seems to move in a spiral, and the prospects of life and work returning to the way it was before 2020 were dwindling. But if I hoped for some wisdom to take from all we'd withstood in those months, it was to hold on to the essence of the work: two people coming together because of the suffering of one of them, and in the process both becoming changed by it. The job of a GP had been moulded and squeezed out of shape by the intense pressure of these early months of the pandemic, the months I've attempted to chart, but despite it all, the fundamentals of its care work remained the same: see sick people, treat disease, ease suffering.

One by one European countries began to report rising cases, though the death rate of those countries stayed mercifully low for the time being. The US, Brazil and India were all recording terrifying figures for its spread, though even there the 'case fatality rate' seemed to be dropping, although whether this was because the virus itself was mutating or because the groups most affected were too young for the most fatal outcomes of the virus, wasn't yet clear. In the UK, Manchester and York went back under a variation of lockdown: no family groups could meet in one another's houses, even in the gardens, though pubs remained open; cinemas and beauty parlours had been due to open for the first time in almost five months, but then they were told they could not.

The papers began to acknowledge a second wave – the number of newly confirmed positive cases in the UK had been rising slowly but steadily through July from 400, to 500, to 800 a day, and by mid-August it had got to 1,000, though the proportion of that figure contributed by Scotland, with a tenth of the population of the UK as a whole, were still tiny.

Back in the convalescent weeks of June there had been predictions that Scotland might be Covid-free by August, but that optimism was revealed as unfounded, even deluded – an outbreak in Aberdeen triggered Scotland's first local lockdown, then a fishing boat carried a spore of it to Orkney where it bloomed into several communities across the archipelago. A frenetic contact-tracing operation managed to bring it under control. I called my friends and colleagues in the islands, knowing how careful all had been in following the guidance, aware of how swiftly the good work of months could be undone.

The threat of going back into the isolation of lockdown had a chilling effect on many of the people I spoke with in my own clinic each day; some who'd arranged foreign holidays changed their plans as soon as it became clear just how insidious and pervasive the threat remained. 'At least we're better prepared now,' said a woman who'd shielded for many months. 'And it can't go on forever – can it?'

In an interview with the novelist Ali Smith, I read of her surprise at the 'unexpected communality' that the pandemic had revealed, of the importance of acknowledging the 'griefwork and transformation that the virus has visited on us all across the country, all across the world'. That griefwork never stopped – from time to time I'd speak with the relatives of those lost to the virus, but the more pressing griefs that first week in August were of the teenagers frustrated by an examination system that had summarily downgraded their results by postcode, and the young professionals who, in rising numbers, were losing their jobs as the economic recession began its axe work. And the transformations that Ali Smith spoke of continued to visit themselves on my profession: I began to suspect that stop-gap measures, like video encounters and telephone triage, were being promoted as an enduring ideological shift.

The suggestion, by email, that I embrace a 'digital first' model of practising medicine by default gave me a jolt. The tone of such directives radiated a conviction that shifting healthcare online would be cheaper but was equally safe – a prediction as without foundation as Scotland being Covid-free by August.

In the GP press many of my colleagues complained of being swamped by online and telephone demands that couldn't be met safely: commercial GP services operating through smartphone applications can only do so because there's an NHS there to *see* the patients who need urgent face to face review. And brushed over by the enthusiasts of tele-medicine was any acknowledgement that distanced medicine had only been possible through these months because it was buttressed by years of personal encounters, by a shared inner register of experience between GP and patient that accepted the difficulties the pandemic had imposed, but was nourished by a time and a relationship when encounters were more straightforward. The video calls I make to a patient in the throes of a panic attack help in part because my face is familiar, as is the backdrop of my office – the patient can see the familiar space on their smartphone, as together we talk and breathe through their peak of anxiety. As time goes on, and if telemedicine prevails, those relationships forged in person will become more remote, and the medicine GPs practise will become more perfunctory, based on the avoidance of being sued rather than on what's best for the patient. Those conversations would be not 'consultations', but triage, fire-fighting, damage limitation.

It's difficult enough to engage with the unique complexity of another human being's suffering in ten or twelve minutes when sharing the same space, but on the telephone it's near impossible. Many colleagues confessed to feeling deep exhaustion after a couple of hours on the phone trying to manage their patients at a distance, as if that effort, and the rapid switching between patients, worked together to augment a constant, lurking suspicion that at best corners were being cut and at worst serious diagnoses were being missed. My own kids picked up a cough after starting back at school, and so, for a couple of days, while we were waiting for their swab result (negative) I was consulting from home – ringing patient after patient, knowing that the prescriptions and letters I typed out were printing in the clinic's back office, twelve miles away, and would have to be signed by my colleagues. Whichever patients I gauged needed to be seen face to face were added to my colleagues' already lengthy clinic lists. It was a fix, but a temporary one – awkward and unpleasant.

I mentioned the drive to 'digital first' to a colleague with indignation. 'Some people just prefer it this way,' he said, 'sitting in their offices, not seeing anyone.'

'Why did they go into medicine, then?' I asked. But he only shrugged.

*

The Edinburgh Access Practice needed me for locum shifts a couple of times a month, and there, too, the clinics had begun to open up – not the twelve appointments of before, but on every shift I'd see at least three people in person and call up to twelve more on the phone. For most, lockdown in a hotel room, bedsit or B&B room hadn't been easy, but the silver lining for that community was that there was hardly anyone left sleeping rough in the city.

A second call came in for volunteers to help with another vaccine trial, this one conducted by Imperial College London. I got in touch with Becky Sutherland to see whether I could be useful. An email arrived asking if I could provide some island cover in Orkney through the winter, and I began to make arrangements for my own practice in Edinburgh, so that I might at least be in a position to help.

The August edition of the *Journal of the Royal College of GPs* arrived: page after page celebrating, lamenting, pleading and arguing about the transformations imposed on the profession. It spoke uneasily of the racial disparities of this disease – the startling statistic that those of black or Asian ethnicity had between double and quadruple the risk of serious complications from Covid-19 of 'white British' people. It detailed, too, the structural racism within the NHS, and recounted one doctor's sickening experience of having a patient refuse his care because of his skin colour. On the letters page anxiety over the mental-health fallout of lockdown was dominant – consultations for stress, depression and anxiety were said to have doubled, induced in part by fear of the virus, but also by poverty, loneliness, unemployment and ailing support services. Many GPs were uneasy about the extent to which their routine work had been shut down by the extraordinary measures taken to protect the health service from the virus.

'One disease should not define the entire health system,' wrote one policy researcher, based in Florida. 'Access to care for conditions other than Covid-19-like illness need not be lost.'

One London GP, James Hibberd, noticed how much our understanding of Covid-19 had evolved since the beginning of the year, but also how its characterisation as a 'disease' had shifted through that period, from a short-term illness of the airways to one of ITU, lung scarring, blood clotting and skin rashes. Then the widely publicised alert that a few children had been stricken by a dangerous autoimmune reaction, and latterly yet another phase, of Covid-19 as a chronic post-viral illness.

In only seven months we'd come a long way in our understanding of how this virus engages and afflicts human beings, but we were still in an early phase of that encounter. Disease is about pathology, but it's also about culture: Hibberd was anxious that, in adopting these different frames of recognition for Covid-19, GPs appreciate that they inevitably emphasise some features at the expense of others. It is important that different kinds of healthcare workers feel able to contribute to the evolution of the disease narrative, and not cede too much to sensational journalism or to super-specialist experiences of the illness that only a tiny proportion of the population will ever suffer. This malleability of the ways in which we experience disease came up in conversation with a friend, who spoke of her grandmother's death from viral pneumonia a couple of years before the pandemic broke. 'At the time it was seen very differently from how I hear about death from Covid-19,' she said. 'There was a lot of talk of it being "the old man's friend", that it was a quick, relatively painless and easy way out from a life that was becoming exhausting and not terribly enjoyable. I think that's what she thought about it as well.'

Through Autumn, with infection rates rising sharply, there was a breakdown in the testing system, particularly in England, where some people who needed a Covid test were being directed hundreds of miles from home, even across the Solent to the Isle of Wight. I was still unable to return to the routine of my pre-pandemic job, the job for which I was trained: a sequence of people coming together in a waiting room and being called through one by one to the privacy of the consulting space, to be asked about their rashes and coughs, anxieties and idiosyncrasies, aches and infections, tumours and troubles. The perennial task of approaching the last patient of the day with as much energy and enthusiasm as the first. Newborn baby checks and contraceptive advice, work stresses and family hang-ups, fevers, limps and sprains, hallucinations and paranoias, fading eyesight and dwindling libidos. The arc of life in plain sight, from its inception to its conclusion.

Instead it had become a job of telephone management, of triage and guesswork, of bringing into the surgery only those with the most worrying of symptoms, or those in the deepest distress. In the out of hours centre I had flashbacks to April. We began to see a steep rise in Covid-19 patients again: feverish, breathless and in need of admission to hospital. And with the receptionists and practice nurses, my colleagues and I began to grapple with the formidable logistics of administering winter flu vaccines in a world where it would be inadvisable to bring together the very people who needed them most. As infection rates continued to climb across the world, the UK began tightening restrictions. A grim milestone was passed: a million 'official' deaths from the virus

– though the true figure was undoubtedly far higher. The US President came down with Covid-19. Students returned to their universities all across the UK and, as predicted, the virus began to spread rapidly through halls of residence. My clinic is just a few hundred yards from one of Edinburgh University's largest halls, and within days of the new semester I was conducting video consultations with new students in locked-down corridors, anxious as well as furious that their university lives were being curtailed before they had even begun.

The Halloween announcement that England would re-enter lockdown for an initial period of four weeks came like a hammer blow – all year I'd seen just how devastating the consequences of restrictions had been, and now we'd have to endure lockdown again, in winter. 'All our batteries are already at twenty per cent,' said a friend. 'If only human beings had a "low power mode".' But among those difficulties there was a glimmer of hope: on 9 November a vaccine trial showed positive early results, and my practice was asked whether we'd help administer it. It would be a huge logistical operation that might commence even before the year's end. On shift in the out of hours centre that weekend there was a notice in the corridor: 'After Covid I'm Going To …', and staff members were asked to stick up Post-it notes with their plans. For the first time, it felt like those plans might come true.

I worked Christmas Day in the out of hours clinic – one of the quietest I've known – but had New Year off to celebrate the end of what had been an atrocious year. Not that there were any parties. The UK government had planned to slacken restrictions for Christmas and allow a three-day free-for-all of nationwide travel. But those ambitious plans had to be curtailed at devastatingly short notice, once it became clear just how quickly case numbers were accelerating. Among my patients I heard of many lonely Christmas dinners, and though some families made extraordinary efforts to see loved ones briefly in the areas of the country where it was permitted, the consequences of the easing of lockdown could also be tragic. Case numbers shot up; one grandfather I heard of, who'd isolated for much of 2020, caught coronavirus from an asymptomatic family member over his Christmas dinner and died right about the time he would have received his first vaccine.

RECOVERY

'I shall conclude the account of this calamitous year
therefore with a coarse but sincere stanza of my own.'
Daniel Defoe
A Journal of the Plague Year

Towards the end of *A Fortunate Man*, John Berger's reflection on the daily work of a general practitioner called John Sassall, Berger speaks of his struggle to bring his thoughts to a conclusion. Any chosen conclusion would be arbitrary, he writes, because 'Sassall is alive and working, and my speculations have paralleled the process of his continuing life – anxious to see the maximum possible, but inevitably half-blind, like an owl in bright daylight. Too blind to see the conclusion for certain, aware only of the alternatives.' Berger felt almost paralysed by the reality of summating a life still in development, evolving and responding to events.

The same could be said of the story I've been telling, which hasn't been one of a single person and his profession, but instead the evolution of a pandemic seen from inside that profession. And as I write, the pandemic goes on, and in my own country is accelerating again. Though it's conceivable that this coronavirus will be eliminated as smallpox was once eliminated, it is more likely that it will become a fact of life – like influenza, like adenovirus, like measles – and, like those other viruses, it will settle into one of many possible diagnoses in the minds of all future doctors and nurses whenever they encounter a sick patient who needs help.

Thankfully clinicians everywhere are at the same time becoming accustomed to treating this virus, and accomplished at recognising its signs and symptoms, its unusual rashes, high fevers, its effect on our sense of smell and taste, and the enduring fatigue that may complicate its convalescence. Even if we never learn how to annihilate it, it's clear that we now have the capacity to quickly generate vaccines that will suppress it.

As Berger struggled in *A Fortunate Man* to weigh up the many factors of the life that he had examined, and the myriad elements of the general practitioner's work, he envisaged his readers' frustration. 'The future has to be problematic,' he imagines one saying. 'Conclude by drawing up the account to date: let it be an admittedly incomplete conclusion.'

As we moved into 2021 the death rates climbed and the lockdown persisted. Schools were closed, and there were at least two other shadow pandemics unfolding. First, that of all the other serious health conditions going unrecognised, because NHS attention had, by necessity, been obliged to focus so much on the virus. Second, GPs were firefighting an explosion in mental-health difficulties – anxiety, addictions, insomnia, depression, self-harm, psychosis – triggered not just by the virus, but by the measures we'd had to take against it. Every day I heard new stories about the strain lockdown puts on kids, on marriages, on those already isolated, and I was witnessing a burgeoning epidemic of loneliness. A typical morning might see three separate consultations for which loneliness was the principle problem – from self-harming students to divorced dads to isolated pensioners taking overdoses. I became accustomed to clinics dominated by mental-health concerns. People were unable to share those aspects of our humanity that help us most in times of distress, and that come most naturally, such as touch, speech, sharing space. I was hopeful that the vaccine rollout would prove an effective antidote to the sense of hopelessness that, for the past few months, had been spreading and deepening among many of my patients.

The staff vaccination programme for NHS Lothian began, and after nine months of feeling intensely exposed every time we assessed coronavirus patients, the feeling of relief was extraordinary: our practice WhatsApp group was taken over by celebratory memes and emojis. As Pfizer was the first vaccine to be approved it would be the one that staff would receive; the first shipment of vials came through to Lothian a day or two later.

My appointment was at nine o'clock sharp the following week. I drove to St John's Hospital in West Lothian through bands of freezing fog, then made my way from the frosted haze of the car park, following a trail of laminated yellow notices to the hospital's top floor. It's a brown-brick, three-level affair built in the 1980s, and the view from the top floor above the fog was clear and luminous. The sun was rising but its orange light was too weak, or the day too cold, for it to effectively clear the air. To the south I could just about make out the pharmaceutical factory in Livingston where a French company, Valneva, had another Covid-19 vaccine in development.

The hospital corridors were quiet, though the wards were filling up with Covid patients; case numbers were racing back towards the worst days of the previous year. By the middle of January there were over 1,200 deaths in the UK *every day* – worse even than the peak of April 2020. Over the course of the pandemic I'd admitted numerous patients to those same wards – each of them breathless and fevered, many of them panic-stricken.

One stands out in memory: an ordinarily healthy 60-year-old man whom I'll call Mr Denison. He lived alone and had been suffering a cough and fever for a week but – nine months into the pandemic – didn't think to book a Covid test. He had carried on going out, seeing his family, catching up with friends. If the lungs are going to be severely affected by coronavirus, it usually happens seven to ten days from the onset of fever. Right on cue, Mr Denison called for a GP home visit on day nine – his breathlessness had become so severe he was struggling to walk to the toilet.

I remember phoning him from the car to ask him to sit by his front door, then standing on his doorstep to put on an apron, doubled gloves and a visor. I nudged open his door to see him sitting on his staircase in a grimy bathrobe. He looked frightened. I stepped in over his threshold, put an oxygen sensor on his finger, and a gloved hand on his shoulder. His breaths came quickly, at nearly thirty a minute, and I arranged an ambulance to take him to St John's. In the subsequent days I followed the course of his admission by logging onto the hospital system: he'd been started on the steroid dexamethasone and a new antiviral drug, and he was making a good recovery. The last entry I saw expressed the hope that he would be well enough to be discharged the following week. Intensive treatment units filled to capacity make the headlines, but it's just as often the slow, bed-bound recoveries necessitated by this disease that were placing such immense pressure on the NHS.

From the vaccine clinic on the top floor of St John's Hospital, looking out over the gathering morning light, it made me happy to think of Mr Denison convalescing next door, enjoying this same view. If he hadn't been in a 'red' restricted Covid ward I would have popped in to say hello. The nurse on duty, Kirsty, checked my name and date of birth, that I didn't have any allergies and that I'd read through the information that had been emailed from the health board. As she drew up the vaccine from a vial I caught a flash of looping, cursive script down her forearm. 'What have you got there?' I asked. She lifted her arm to give me a better view of her tattoo: 'Always Look On The Bright Side Of Life'.

'Seems like a good philosophy,' I said.

She laughed. 'It's the *only* philosophy.' She showed me the vial: a plain little glass jar, labelled in black and white, stamped 'Pfizer BioNTech'. She drew up 0.3 ml into a fine-gauge syringe, and turned to me. 'Left or right arm?'

'Go with the left,' I said. 'In case it's a sore one.' The familiar spike, an electric jangle of cold liquid infiltrating muscle, and we were done. 'Just take a seat next door for ten minutes or so,' she said. 'We don't want you having an anaphylaxis halfway down the corridor.' On the syringe tray I saw that she had two vials of adrenaline drawn up and ready to go, just in case.

By late January nearly every care home resident in Lothian had been offered a first dose, as had the healthcare workers, and we began to plan the first-dose vaccination of all the over-80s. For my small practice, that was about 140 people. Lists were drawn up, clinics rearranged – a huge effort on behalf of the receptionists and the practice manager, all choreographed to make sure there would never be more than four in the waiting room. All we needed was a supply of the vaccine. Priority was given to those practices with large populations of over-80s, and my own was near the back of the queue.

All of my GP colleagues had signed up to work in Edinburgh's Mass Vaccination Centres, and it was impressive to see crowds of nurses, optometrists, dentists and doctors offer their weekends and days off to the national effort. NHS managers too – the speed at which they had moved both nationally and regionally had been formidable; it was thanks to them, as well as the foresight of those who had invested in and pre-ordered millions of doses, that the UK was among the fastest to roll out vaccination anywhere in the world. The schools had been closed since Christmas which meant I was limited in the shifts I could offer, as the days I wasn't in clinic I needed to be home-schooling my kids.

In late January I left Edinburgh again for the Orkney Islands to spend a week standing in for one of the nurse practitioners on an island with a population of just 300 and, thankfully, no coronavirus. It was a six-hour drive to the ferry terminal along empty roads, passing highway signs that still read 'Stay Home, Protect the NHS, Save Lives'. It was maddening to think that the UK had been so lax in policing quarantine, and so disorganised in terms of testing and tracing, that this third lockdown had become necessary. All travel to the islands was still closed, except to essential workers. At the ferry office I produced the letter confirming that I was going to work for NHS Orkney, and was allowed to join a queue that consisted of just one other car. Storm Christoph was incoming, and for the 90-minute crossing I lay along a seat in the empty lounge being hoisted and dropped as if I lay in a rowing boat, not a vessel of 9,000 tons.

It was a week of blizzards, and though I always carried an on-call bleep, the clinics I conducted were of just three or four consultations a day – it felt like a treat to have so much time with patients. Although I had no symptoms and had been vaccinated, each one was assessed from behind a mask and gloves on the off chance I could be transmitting the virus. Every lunchtime there were home visits in my dual role as the substitute district nurse, and on my rounds I heard story after story of how well Orkney, and in particular its smaller isles, had been protected – as indeed any island has had the potential to protect itself from the pandemic by controlling and quarantining arrivals. It was a relief that Orkney had completed the first round of vaccination for all the over-80s just before I had arrived, a full fortnight before my own patients in Edinburgh would receive it.

It's a much joked-about law within medicine, at least in Scotland, that anyone arriving for vaccination must remove at least three layers of clothing before we can get at their arm (those who turn up in a vest under one thick overcoat – we salute you). But in truth I don't really mind the delays caused by the removal of clothing – it opens up the possibility of conversation. One of the first vaccinations I gave back at my clinic in Edinburgh was to a proud, quiet man in his mid-eighties; we hadn't met since April 2020, when his wife died of Covid-19. As he slowly removed his hat, scarf, jacket, pullover, then began painstakingly to roll up his shirt sleeve, we talked about the loneliness of this year; how sad he has been not seeing his great-grandchildren; the dismal, restricted funeral he'd had for his wife. He didn't show any anger over her death, only sorrow. As I vaccinated him against the disease that killed her, he uttered a solemn, heartfelt thanks.

A vaccine consultation consists of just a couple of questions, an enquiry about allergies, then a syringe is drawn up with some clear fluid from a glass vial, and, seconds later pushed into an arm, sinking it into muscle tissue at a depth of a centimetre or so. The precise location in the muscle doesn't really matter. Needle binned, a sticking plaster if it bleeds, and you're done. It's about the simplest medical encounter it's possible to have, though among the most transformative.

One by one, the over-80s began to trickle into our waiting room, relief on their faces, gratitude, as well as a kind of questioning disbelief: Is this really going to free us? Some patients I hadn't seen since March; the oldest was 95, and the youngest 79. Among many encounters, I remember one woman asking me if this was really the best use of the vaccines.

'What do you mean?' I asked.

'All us old folks, doing us first. Shouldn't you be doing the teachers?'

I smiled at her generosity of spirit. 'It's not up to me,' I said. 'Now roll up your sleeve!'

Only one of my elderly patients declined, despite my reassurances. If she caught Covid as a consequence of that refusal I knew my colleagues would of course do everything they could to help her. Her arguments against immunisation were spangled with groundless conspiracy theories picked up on Facebook, and made me think of something the great Canadian physician, William Osler, wrote of anti-vaxxers a century ago:

> I will go into the next severe epidemic with ten selected, vaccinated persons and ten selected, unvaccinated persons – I should prefer to choose the latter – three members of Parliament, three anti-vaccination doctors (if they can be found), and four anti-vaccination propagandists. And I will make this promise – neither to jeer nor jibe when they catch the disease, but to look after them as brothers, and for the four or five who are certain to die, I will try to arrange the funerals with all the pomp and ceremony of an anti-vaccination demonstration.*

---

* William Osler, *Man's Redemption of Man* (New York, Hoeber, 1915) p. 46–7.

Covid-19 had been so excruciatingly difficult to manage because it takes three to four weeks to gauge the effects of any intervention. But through the spring of 2021, as a consequence of the gathering pace of vaccination, we saw hospitalisations fall, and fall, and fall, despite the easing of lockdown restrictions. Even when vaccination didn't seem to prevent *infection*, it had a tremendous effect on diminishing the severity of the disease, so that hospital was rarely needed. A 95-year old friend of my family – a woman who babysat for me as a boy – proved the rule, catching Covid three weeks after her first dose. With her age and frailty she was at significant risk, but developed only a cough and a mild fever.

That remained the greatest hope: that even if it proves impossible to eliminate SARS-CoV2 from the population, and even if recurrent iterations of vaccine won't entirely prevent infection with new variants of the virus, the dangers of that infection will be mitigated, fatal outcomes will be averted, and society can slowly begin to open up. Transmission will rise, but hospitals won't be overwhelmed. The immense mental-health and social and economic benefits of opening up still have to be balanced against significant risks – death from Covid among the under-50s is relatively rare, but it can still be a terrible, terrifying disease, capable of rendering its victims breathless and exhausted for weeks (and in some cases, months), long after its fevers have run their course. In March 2021 a study in *Nature Medicine* estimated that around 13 per cent of sufferers have symptoms lasting longer than four weeks, and 2 per cent still have symptoms at three months – most commonly fatigue, headache, breathlessness and loss of smell.*

Homeless people in Edinburgh have a life expectancy in

---

* Sudre, C.H., Murray, B., Varsavsky, T. et al., 'Attributes and predictors of long COVID', *Nature Medicine* 27, 626–31 (2021).

the mid-forties – worse than the residents of Gaza (52) or Chad (54). Much had been learned in how to protect such a vulnerable population, and a new hotel towards the West End of the city had taken over as a night shelter. The Access Practice was stocked with Covid vaccines so that on duty there I was able to offer the jab to patients with no fixed address as they came through. On my first shift at one of the mass vaccination centres I turned up to see neat, ordered cubicles, ubiquitous NHS branding, smiling, cheerful colleagues and most importantly, fridges filled with Covid-19 vaccine. After a year of social distancing, it was joyous, welcome and faintly surreal to be again in a space designed for the mass congregation of human beings. The numbers to be vaccinated were daunting, but there was a spirit of anticipation and celebration in the air.

Opening my first box of vials there in anticipation of the queues of people eager to take this step towards getting our lives back to normal, I thought of a friend in Orkney, a GP who'd already vaccinated all the over-80s of his practice, and who'd begun to call in the over-70s. We met briefly in Kirkwall, outdoors, on my journey from Orkney back to Edinburgh. 'How did it feel to get started?' I asked him.

'I almost wept as I opened that box of vials,' he said, smiling at the memory. 'Each one was hope – pure, liquid hope.'

On my bicycle, pedalling to and from my medical practice, I saw the swans at the canal had a new brood of cygnets – five this year. It was that, more than the newspaper headlines, which made me realise how long we'd been coping with this pandemic, and how long we might still have to endure. The seasons were passing; one by one the restrictions on shops, pubs, restaurants, gatherings, began to fall away, but for most of my patients it was an edgy, nervous re-opening – images from a third wave in India, as bad as anything seen earlier in the pandemic, and the arrival of new, more transmissible variants of the virus, subdued many celebrations. It was clear the quarantine system was not working as it should. By June nearly everyone over 30 in the UK had been offered at least one dose, and hospitalisation rates had plummeted from a peak of 4,500 *per day* across the UK in early January to around 100 – there were frequent days when, across Scotland, no-one at all was admitted to hospital with Covid-19, and no-one died of it. April 2020 had seen the first peak of virus transmission and deaths, then January 2021 had seen another. With the arrival of a new, highly transmissible 'Delta' variant, infection rates climbed through June, and I watched the hospitalisation rates with anxiety, hoping they'd stay low – which they seemed to do in the UK. Summery weather, and the renewed possibilities of holidays, meant an improvement in mental health for many of my patients even as transmission climbed. It was safer not to hope for any return to 'normality' – as the weeks turned into months, it was clear we'd emerge from this pandemic not into the world as it was before, but into a new, wiser and more cautious one.

It felt like society, and the profession I love, was in slow recovery, but it would be a lengthy convalescence. Through June the virus continued to spread rapidly in the UK, and though hospitalisation rates and death rates at first remained low, by July these too had begun to rise (though at nothing like the levels seen in the first or second waves). At the weekend and evening service almost all the patients I assessed with debilitating Covid-19 were those who had turned down the offer of a vaccine. By mid-July, as four million deaths worldwide were recorded and three and a half billion doses of vaccine had been delivered, the UK's prime minister announced the repeal of almost all restrictions on social gatherings. It was tempting to think of the pandemic as coming to an end, but it was clear that both locally and globally that was far from the case. The Director-General of the WHO called for greater investment by rich countries in vaccine provision for the poor. 'It's time to move beyond the cycle of panic and invest in equitable health systems and the global health architecture,' he said. 'At the core of all of our efforts must be health for all, based on strong primary healthcare.' Doctors and nurses who worked within their communities were, he said, 'the cornerstone of social, economic and political stability.'

Edinburgh University's Futures Institute, a body set up to promote interdisciplinary scholarship, asked if I'd give a talk with England's Chief Medical Officer, Chris Whitty, on the opportunities the pandemic might offer to rethink how, as a society, we offer care. I began by speaking of how poverty and deprivation doubled your chances of death from coronavirus, but that because of the pandemic we'd made a tentative start at solving one of the most intractable of society's problems – homelessness. I spoke of the immense difficulties that lockdowns impose on us as social, gregarious beings, of the sacrifices that had been made by the young on behalf of the old. I moved on to speak of pride in the NHS, and in my colleagues in medicine, nursing and caring, as well as how inspirational it had been to see the way professionals had been allowed to get on and solve immense challenges like vaccine development, the acceleration of digital healthcare, the restructuring of our clinics and hospitals and mass public vaccination.

The seismic shock of the virus had opened up cracks in our society, and we had a responsibility to do more than just paper over those cracks. 'Recovery' comes from a root meaning 'to regain consciousness', and the pandemic had made us acutely conscious of how interconnected and interdependent we are as human beings, and how vital and undervalued the work of caring is. No one's safe until we're all safe. 'Convalescence' derives from a word meaning 'to grow in strength', and I hoped that society as well as the caring professions would ultimately prove stronger for the ordeal.

Though many new doctors still swear by the Hippocratic Oath, the medicine practised today is unrecognisable from that practised 2,500 years ago in Greece. The aim of the Edinburgh Futures Institute was to promote dialogue between the arts and the sciences, and so I concluded my hopes for the future with a poem by James Robertson, commissioned during that terrible year of 2020 for the Royal College of Physicians of Edinburgh. The poem, 'Hippocrates in Queen Street', was presented to an outgoing president, Derek Bell, and was framed as a soliloquy addressed by that old Greek physician to those of us trying to practise it in the cold Athens of the north. It was in Queen Street's old college library that I had begun writing up this account.

Robertson invoked three ancient, mythical symbols of medicine: the snake that winds around the staff of Aesculapius, the centaur Chiron (who taught medicine to mankind), and a cockerel of light. Like the best poetry, it offers a series of truths, elegantly compressed and distilled. The poem acts as a reminder that the work of medicine is without end, but Robertson's words also charge me with the hope that the core of medicine – the clinical encounter, with its alliance of science, kindness and intensive care – will endure, and that humanity will recover from this pandemic, as it has from so many in the past:

Your patient is your mirror: therefore, look with
     sympathy;
work with the faults and flaws, see the stories in the
     scars,

replace what worn-out parts can be replaced and,
when remedy cannot be found, in the last resort be
    kind.
The world needs all the kindness it can get.
Our time is short. The snake casts off its skin;
the cockerel calls up the morning light;
we glimpse the centaur leaping in the wood;
we work, we live, we love; we say good night.

But not just yet. Although *I* will now disappear,
life is what *you* are for, and why you are here.

Edinburgh, July 2021

THANKS

to my colleagues, many of whom have devoted far more hours to direct patient care through this pandemic than I have. There are scores of them deserving of thanks, but special mention must be made of Andrew Watson, Angela Colburn-Veitch, Anne Nicolson, Bean Dhaun, Becky Sutherland, Carey Lunan, Cathy Grant, Charlie Siderfin, Claire Gordon, Claudia Galante, Colin Speight, Digby Thomas, Eileen Sanderson, Fiona Wright, Gareth Evans, Geraldine Fraser, Helen Britton, Ishbel White, Janis Blair, Jenna Pemberton, John Budd, Justin Perry, Karen Stevenson, Kate Megaw, Laura Muir, Lesley Dawson, Lynsay McDonald, Michaela Johnson, Mimi Cogliano, Nicola Gray, Peter D orward, Rankin Barr, Sharon Lawson, Sheila Ross, Sian Tucker, Tina Brown and Wojtek Wojcik.

It often feels as if I have two sides to my mind and my life: medicine and writing work together like the left and right feet of a steady gait, or the left and right eyes that give depth to vision. Thanks are due also to my colleagues over on the other side, at Profile Books. We'd never worked on a book together quite like this one; the trust and confidence shown by Cecily Gayford and Andrew Franklin has been immense, and immensely appreciated. Thanks also to Graeme Hall, Penny Daniel, Valentina Zanca, Flora Willis, Peter Dyer, Jack Smyth, Sally Holloway, Fran Fabriczki and Lottie Fyfe at Profile, and to Clare Longrigg and David Wolf who first commissioned me to write about the pandemic as seen from the community, for Long Reads in the *Guardian* in March and May 2020, and February 2021. I'm indebted to the genius of James Robertson, and to his generosity in permitting me to quote from 'Hippocrates in Queen Street'. To my agent Jenny Brown for all the coffee, cake, and putting up with me all these years. And finally, much gratitude and love to Esa.